Dr. Irma I. Sierra

BEYOND THE
POWER OF THE
MAGNET

Beyond the Power of the Magnet © Irma I. Sierra, 2023
Independent Publication by Dr. Irma Sierra, LLC, 2025
All Rights Reserved. San Juan, Puerto Rico.

ISBN: 979-8-9985898-1-2
www.irmasierra.com

Original Editorial Management: Yasmín Rodríguez
Translation: Marieli A. De J. Gordils
Self-publishing consultancy & Book Production:
The Writing Ghost®, Inc.
www.thewritingghost.com

Cover Design: Gil Acosta Design
www.gilacosta.com

Author's Photos: Raúl Romero Photography
raulromerophotography@gmail.com

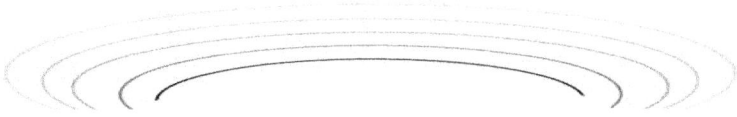

Dedication

For my grandchildren and future generations:

I hope this collection of knowledge resonates deeply within you and that your thirst for information becomes an unwavering tool in your lives.

May you benefit from the power of magnetic energy and the therapeutic properties of magnets.

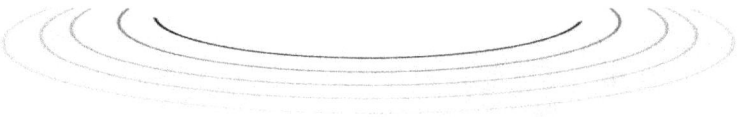

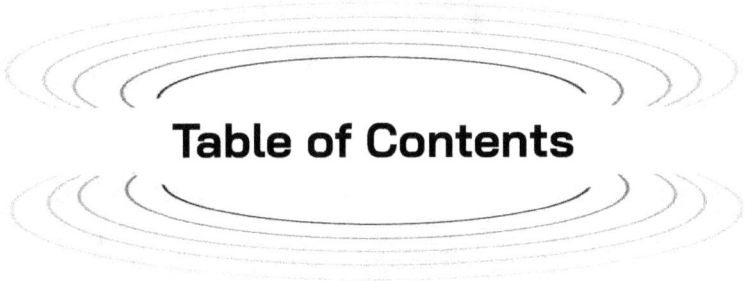

Table of Contents

Acknowledgments

I want to express my heartfelt gratitude to my husband, Jorge—my best friend—who has always stood by my side, holding my hand through this journey. To my children, Jorge, Adrián, and Alexandra: you are my inspiration, and I will forever be grateful for all of you. Each day, you make me prouder than the last. Thank you for always being there from the very beginning and for joining me in helping others through the power of magnets!

I am deeply grateful to my parents for believing in me and allowing me to venture into the world and pursue this career at just seventeen years old. They truly deserve an award for trusting me at a time when making a phone call still required a quarter and an operator. Thank you for your unconditional love!

To all my team at *Health Magnetic Store & More,* who share my dream of spreading awareness about magnetic devices and the importance of living a magnetic life, thank you! To my readers, patients, and clients, whose interest in my work continues to inspire me, I am profoundly grateful. Thank you for opening your hearts and minds a little more each day.

And to God, my universe and my source of life, I am infinitely GRATEFUL!

Another Book About Magnets? Why?

You might be wondering: why another book about magnets? What makes this one any different? It's a fair question, especially considering that *Power in a Magnet*, published in 2007, remains relevant today, standing the test of time with its trustworthy and enduring information. Good science always endures.

Although there is already an abundance of excellent information on magnets, biomagnetism, and their relationship to human health, this book aims to empower its readers to benefit from this science while offering a fresh perspective on the discipline.

In simple terms, biomagnetism refers to the effects of energy from a magnet's static or pulsating magnetic field on biological systems. Throughout these pages, we will explore everything that statement entails.

I consider myself incredibly fortunate to be the daughter of Dr. Ralph U. Sierra, the first Puerto Rican to introduce chiropractic care to Puerto Rico. What a fascinating life we've led! My family has been immersed in chiropractic care since 1948, when my father pioneered its practice on the island. (Although it wasn't until 1952 that he was able to officially register it as a profession in Puerto Rico.) His knowledge, discoveries, and insatiable curiosity have given me a unique perspective, not only on the history of biomagnetism and its lessons but also on its application, development, and benefits for the human body, all backed by science.

Within this book, you will find the story of the rebirth of biomagnetism and the pivotal role my father played in it, along with the fascinating history behind this beneficial and healing science.

Additionally, it serves as a practical guide, introducing techniques I've developed to help you integrate this therapy into your daily life. **You will also discover a wealth of information in a guide full of my own techniques, designed to help you achieve a healthier, more sustainable lifestyle through the unmatched power of magnets.** Finally, this book includes interviews, letters, and invaluable insights from my father, Dr. Ralph U. Sierra, who was the first disciple of Albert Roy Davis, the man widely regarded as the father of biomagnetism as we know it today.

The relationship between Dr. Ralph U. Sierra and Dr. Albert Roy Davis was a collaboration between two scientists committed to continuous growth and well-being. It was also the catalyst for the advancement of this discipline. In my opinion, what truly popularized biomagnetism among health professionals in the United States was my father's remarkable recovery. He suffered from Ménière's disease (a disorder affecting the inner ear) and prostate inflammation, yet he fully healed by applying Dr. Davis' teachings without the need for surgery.

My childhood coincided with the rising popularity of chiropractic care and biomagnetism in Puerto Rico. Long before I was born, Dr. Sierra regularly visited the Children's Hospital (*Hospital del Niño*) in San Juan to provide pediatric chiropractic treatments. Before he even founded the Puerto Rico Science Research Laboratory, I became his first pediatric patient treated with magnets. He treated me, our family, and our friends while compiling research and expanding his scientific knowledge.

To me, his laboratory was a magical place, where I witnessed his groundbreaking research and treatments, particularly in musculoskeletal conditions, joint disorders, arthritis, and even cancer. He also studied the effects of biomagnetism on seed biology and plant growth. Over the years, he helped many athletes and individuals who had lost all hope of finding relief. Witnessing his work fueled my own curiosity and passion for this field.

So, what makes this book special? It's not just about inspiring readers to pursue better health. It also tells the story of two scientists who propelled a science that my family and I continue to keep alive today.

My heritage is deeply intertwined with my mission to improve my patients' quality of life while offering hope to those who believe they've tried everything without success.

My experience with biomagnetism is truly unique. I don't know if there is anyone else in the world who has been using magnets since childhood or who has been continuously exposed to static and pulsating magnetic fields for over fifty consecutive years. I can confidently affirm that, when used correctly, magnets have no negative or harmful effects on overall health or the human body. On the contrary, they help maintain the strength and vitality needed in today's demanding world.

My expertise in this field comes from a lifetime of daily, firsthand experience. I was raised among magnets and magnetic fields from a young age. I have personally witnessed their benefits and healing properties. Even my jewelry is magnetic, and I never take it off. And when I say never, I mean it: I wear it to the beach, in the shower, and even while I sleep. My continuous exposure, combined with my knowledge and practice, provides me with a rare and valuable perspective on this subject.

Now, let's explore the power of the magnet together!

Biomagnetism

Have you ever touched a metallic object and felt a sudden but brief electric shock? This reaction occurs due to the natural energy our bodies generate. As human beings, we contain electricity, energy, and frequencies that inevitably interact with the outside world and with each other within our bodies. But what if we could harness that energy and use it to heal ourselves? This question intrigued scientists and doctors for decades, and among them was my father. The answer to that question is biomagnetism.

Biomagnetism first emerged in San Juan, Puerto Rico, in 1967, thanks to my father, Dr. Ralph U. Sierra. He suffered from Ménière's disease, a condition that primarily affects the inner ear, causing extreme dizziness and hearing loss. He also struggled with an inflamed prostate. In his search for a noninvasive, natural treatment that would help alleviate his symptoms, my father began learning more about biomagnetics. He conducted experiments on himself and met the acclaimed and knowledgeable practitioner of biomagnetics, Albert Roy Davis, in the process.

Because of his relentless pursuit of knowledge and commitment to continuous growth, Dr. Ralph U. Sierra played a pivotal role in introducing both chiropractic care and biomagnetism to Puerto Rico.

Biomagnetism is a scientific and therapeutic approach to wellness that differs from traditional medicine, homeopathy, herbal remedies, and other natural therapies, yet it is fully compatible with both conventional and alternative treatments. This discipline focuses on the effects of magnetic fields on biological systems.

At its core, biomagnetism harnesses the opposing poles of magnets, classified as north (negative energy) and south (positive energy). When applied to specific areas of the body, based on the individual's condition and the ailment being treated, these magnets generate energy that can have beneficial effects.

It is important to clarify that biomagnetism does not seek to replace medical treatments or professional healthcare advice. Rather, it is an internationally recognized therapeutic approach aimed at achieving bioenergetic balance within the body. This balance, known as homeostasis, represents the body's natural state of equilibrium, where all organs and functions operate in harmony (*NCI Dictionaries, n.d.*). Unlike many conventional treatments, biomagnetism is non-invasive and free from side effects, making it a safe and effective alternative.

For decades, scientists, doctors, and scholars worldwide have dedicated themselves to studying the healing benefits of biomagnetism. Dr. Ralph U. Sierra and Albert Roy Davis were among those pioneers, and thanks to their research, we can now experience the advantages of their discoveries. Although there is an extensive body of literature and numerous studies on the benefits of biomagnetism, it remains an underexplored and underutilized field in mainstream medicine.

Studies on the effects of biomagnetism are not limited to its healing potential. The benefits of biomagnetism extend into various fields, including electronics, aerodynamics, and even astronomy.

Another crucial aspect of life on Earth that biomagnetism helps us better understand is the relationship between human beings and the atmosphere. Decades ago, through his research and practice, Ralph U. Sierra demonstrated that solar activity interferes with human frequencies. More recently, researchers have further explored this connection, finding that the frequency of strokes and heart attacks is closely linked to solar activity (Montero Vega et al., 2014). The sun's influence on human biology is so profound that even birth rates increase when solar surface activity fluctuates (Skjærvø et al., 2015). This information suggests the possibility that other celestial bodies in our solar system might also exert an influence on human health.

Just as magnetic poles interact with each other, energy circulates throughout the universe, affecting our biology in both positive and negative ways.

> As you can see, we exist under the constant influence of magnetic fields, and our bodies respond naturally to them starting at the cellular level, the smallest building blocks of life.

Each cell in the human body functions as a tiny electric battery. Scientific data confirms that all living cells, whether from animals or plants, contain positive (south) energy at their nucleus and negative (north) energy within the surrounding protoplasm (Alberts B et al., 2002). This classification defines all human cells as dipolar. Anatomy teaches us that each cell is interconnected through delicate nervous tissue, allowing them to merge and form the organs and systems that sustain life.

Biomagnetism takes this understanding further, revealing that this "subtle nervous tissue" is, in reality, a magnetic field that enables our biology to connect not only with itself but also with the universe we inhabit. These magnetic connections travel at the speed of light so rapidly that they make the nervous system's signals seem slow in comparison. This discovery confirms that cellular physiology can be stimulated or inhibited by magnetic waves generated by a magnet.

The functions of various organs, including the lungs, colon, stomach, pancreas, prostate, uterus, cervix, bones, and human tissue, are fundamentally electrochemical in nature. Based on this knowledge, we can conclude that correctly applying electromagnetic energy to an affected area can not only alleviate certain conditions but, in some cases, even provide a permanent cure. Biomagnetism may hold the key to unlocking solutions for numerous diseases that continue to challenge medical experts worldwide.

Why do I continue emphasizing the importance of a magnet's polarity? While biomagnetism is a highly effective treatment, incorrect application can be more harmful than beneficial. It is crucial to understand the effects each magnetic pole has on the body before using them.

The waves emitted by the north (negative) pole consist of alkaline negative energy, which interrupts and inhibits growth. In contrast, the waves from the south (positive) pole consist of acidic positive energy, which stimulates growth and propagation.

Negative magnetic energy from the north pole reduces acidity, pain, and inflammation. It is commonly used to treat conditions such as cancer, tumors, arthritis, and other illnesses associated with abnormal growths. On the other hand, the positive magnetic energy from the south pole is used to stimulate hair growth, revitalize tired cells. It helps coat and strengthen broken bone segments, assisting in the healing process. Additionally, this energy soothes the nervous system, reducing pain and alleviating stress-induced bone fractures.

However, the south (positive) pole should always be used with caution. In at least 90% of cases, this energy is not recommended because it promotes the growth of harmful organisms. If a patient has a bacterial infection, a virus, or inflammation, applying the positive pole could worsen the condition. Furthermore, practitioners must be careful not to direct the positive south pole's energy toward themselves, as it can be just as detrimental.

> The positive south pole is identified with the color red. Think of the universal red "stop" symbol. Meanwhile, the negative north pole is associated with blue or green, representing a signal to "go" or continue safely.

Once magnets interact with the body, they immediately alter the blood's chemistry. The more frequently the therapy is applied with the correct polarity and intensity, the better the body's biomagnetic energy will function, from the atomic level to the skin. The foundation of the universe and of a healthy life is electronic and natural.

My Story

To share who I am and what I have achieved in life and in the field of biomagnetism, I must first tell you about my parents, Irma Rivera and Dr. Ralph U. Sierra. I am the daughter of extraordinary individuals, and I live my life proud of the legacy they entrusted to me, of the way they raised me and the role they played in shaping the woman, mother, and professional I am today.

Dr. Ralph U. Sierra, a chiropractor, met Irma Rivera sometime after a divorce that had left him emotionally drained. Irma was an executive secretary at the Puerto Rico Electric Power Authority. At one point, she injured her back, and her sister Carmen took her to see Dr. Sierra. After a few adjustments, my father surprised her on one of her visits with tickets to see the opera *Madame Butterfly*. From then on, they were inseparable. My mother left her job to become my father's right hand. Although there was a twenty-three-year age gap between them, they complemented each other perfectly. When my father was fifty-seven years old, I was born. I inherited my mother's joyful spirit and my father's passion for chiropractic, the best of both worlds. I loved spending time with them. We were a very close family. My mom and I were best friends, and my dad and I were partners in crime.

Growing up with a father who essentially pioneered an entirely new branch of healthcare in Puerto Rico was as fascinating as you might imagine. For me, it was normal life, one filled with love and happiness. We always cared for ourselves using homeopathic and holistic methods. There wasn't a single ailment my father couldn't address with an adjustment or magnets, and many people outside our family can attest to that. Whenever someone had a health concern, my father always found a solution that didn't rely solely on modern medicine.

As a child, I was very thin and small because I didn't like to eat. How did my dad handle that? With iron and vitamin injections to keep me nourished. That was just how things worked at home. Even so, I hardly remember ever getting sick. And when I did, it never lasted long.

> I have a strong immune system, and I'm certain it's not by chance. It's the result of my lifelong commitment to wellness centered on natural ways to support the body. These paths to well-being are available to all of us if we are willing to learn.

Health in our home was always tied to chiropractic care. I was raised with regular adjustments, vitamins, healthy eating habits, natural honey, holistic medicine, and of course, the power of magnets. I didn't find anything unusual about how I was raised, though to others it seemed strange and unconventional. I lived in a state of well-being long before the term became trendy.

Holistic medicine worked so well for me that I was never vaccinated as a child, and I've maintained that choice to this day. My family never thought it was necessary, and I never felt it was essential in adulthood, even as a mother. I did have my tonsils removed at age ten, at the insistence of my maternal aunt. I don't blame her. She had only the best intentions for her niece. After the surgery, I would sometimes soothe the discomfort by wearing a magnetic neck wrap turned toward my throat. That said, I always went to the dentist voluntarily, and had my first bloodwork done when I became pregnant.

I want to make it clear, dear reader, that my life story is not intended as a critique of any healthcare protocols. **I strongly encourage everyone to research, ask questions, and make informed decisions about their health.** Speak with medical professionals, seek knowledge, and never feel pressured to follow a particular standard.

Around the age of fourteen, I became more interested in my father's work as a chiropractor. Beyond just getting adjustments at home, the more I learned about what he did, the more curious I became and the more I wanted to understand. When I told him that I wanted to follow in his footsteps, he immediately began involving me in everything he could, ensuring I actively learned from him. This led me to adopt certain positive habits I saw in his daily routine.

I started eating the same foods he ate. My father loved salads, so I began eating salads. We were highly conscious of our bread and yeast intake, only eating bread that was well-toasted and dry. I adopted most, if not all, of his dietary habits. When he stopped eating meat, I stopped also. He never drank soda or processed juice, so I eliminated them from my diet. He favored a heavier lunch and a lighter dinner, so I followed suit. He also practiced intermittent fasting, and I got used to fasting alongside him. By the late 1950s and early 1960s, my father owned a natural products store in Puerto Rico, where he provided his customers with a variety of health foods and supplements, including freshly squeezed acerola juice.

He was also very physically active. He knew the winning combination for staying healthy was good nutrition and consistent physical activity. In the afternoons, he taught calisthenics at the YMCA. I would go with him and work out too. I learned yoga and developed a habit of always staying in motion.

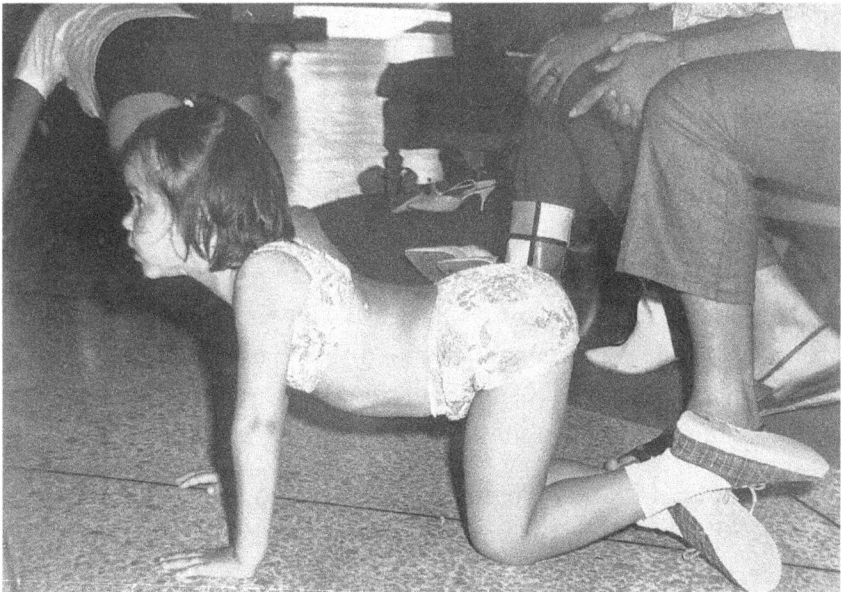

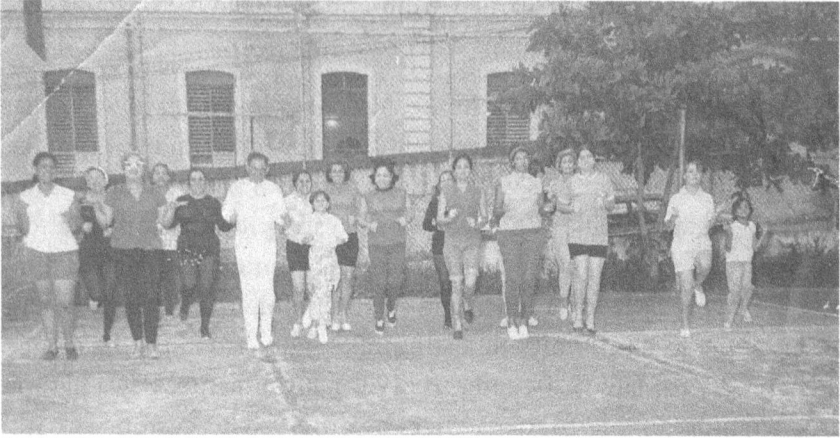

Every morning at 6:30, while I waited for the bus to school, my father would read me my astrological forecast for Gemini. That simple ritual played a role in shaping me into a morning person. I was raised in an environment where positive thinking was encouraged, and the mind-body connection was deeply respected. My father didn't just empha-size a healthy physical routine. He also nurtured the mind and spirit. He taught me to keep a journal, to write down my goals and every-thing I wanted to achieve, always with an end date. He believed this practice would help me visualize my aspirations and learn to love my thoughts, my creations, and everything that made me *Irma*.

Eventually, my parents bought a house where my father established his office, practice, and laboratory. Coincidentally, my future husband's parents would later move just two houses down that very street, but that's a story for later. It was in that home that my father immersed himself in the world of biomagnetics, validating Albert Roy Davis' theories on rats, treating baseball players and his family. As his methods proved increasingly successful, the media took notice. He began re-ceiving interview requests and invitations to share his knowledge at seminars across the globe.

Each summer, my father would close his clinic to travel and lecture. Since these trips coincided with my school break, I accompanied him everywhere. We traveled to Dallas, Los Angeles, Canada, New York, Miami, Mexico, and Trinidad & Tobago. I also saw him lecture at universities in San Juan and Mayagüez on how to create magnetic water for spraying fruits and vegetables. The last conference I attended with him was in St. Louis. That day, as I watched him deliver his lecture, he reminded me of Albert Einstein. That impression, that connection my mind made between the two of them, is something I'll never forget. My dad was my favorite genius.

He was my mentor and the only person who guided me in the fields of biomagnetism and chiropractic care. A fundamental part of my upbringing was learning that magnetism is one of the four fundamental forces of nature, alongside gravity, nuclear energy, and radioactivity. My father taught me that electromagnetism is conceptually equivalent to Qi in ancient Chinese medicine, or prana in other traditions, both meaning "the source of life."

My dad used the planets to explain biomagnetism. At night, we would sit outside, gazing at the sky, as he described how space holds an infinite number of stars and planets, each moving at precise speeds and maintaining specific distances due to an invisible force that preserves the natural order. He would say that our bodies are like miniature universes. Our atoms, molecules, cells, tissues, and organs are magnetic and interconnected, mirroring the cosmos. There exists a natural harmony, a universal intelligence that flows within us without interruption.

Through these lessons, he taught me that human beings are inherently magnetic. If we learn to harness that magnetism, we can channel our own physical and mental healing relying on the tools that nature and the universe already provide. At the time, there was little scientific research, few established procedures, and almost no technological tools to support my father's theories.

Today, however, we have devices like the squid (superconducting quantum interference device), a magnetometer capable of detecting magnetic fields in the brain, heart, and muscles. These human bioenergetic fields can extend as far as fifteen feet around us. My father didn't live to see this, but I'm sure he would have celebrated it.

All this knowledge about magnetism and its connection to human health led me to fully immerse myself in the fields of chiropractic care and biomagnetism. During my senior year of high school, I enrolled in an advanced physics class. For my final project, I wrote an essay in English titled *Magnetism: Its Powers and Effects*. I received a perfect score, and my father was so proud that he had it printed. *"This is your first publication, your first book,"* he told me. I still have copies of it! My teacher was so impressed that he arranged a field trip to my father's lab, and from that point on, my classmates affectionately called me "Magnetita". Magnetita drove the "Magnetomobile" and had a deep passion for her future career in magnetic therapy.

At seventeen, I left Puerto Rico to pursue a chiropractic degree in Long Island, New York, at the State University of New York. While studying there, I got to see my father speak once again, this time at a Silva Mind Control convention. He was incredible. I always tried to be close to him, not only because he was my mentor, but because I had a deep admiration for him as a scientist and as a human being.

During a school break in my second year, I traveled home to visit family. My dad was supposed to pick me up from the airport, but instead, my niece showed up with bad news. She told me that my father had fallen. He was home, but he'd even had to go to the hospital. My mom hadn't told me earlier because she didn't want to stress me out during finals. I understood her reasoning, but it still hurt to be completely unaware of his condition. That's how close we were.

Dr. Ralph U. Sierra was a remarkably determined man. After his fall, he reached out to Albert Roy Davis through letters (which you'll find later in this book!) and carried on as if nothing had happened. But time takes its toll, and by seventy-six, he needed more rest. By that point, we already knew about his prostate condition. I thought it was under control, but later I connected the dots and realized that even though it was managed, **his constant exposure to the south pole of the magnet while giving therapy had likely made things worse.**

When I transferred to the University of Puerto Rico for one semester before starting at the New York Chiropractic College in Long Island, I got one last chance to see him in his lab. I was nineteen. He wasn't doing chiropractic adjustments anymore, but he was still conducting research on biomagnetism. That fall, I began chiropractic school. A year later, my father passed away. He never saw me graduate or practice the profession he had devoted his life to, and which I loved because of him.

My mother was devastated by his passing. They had loved each other so deeply. Any time she tried to speak about him, she would collapse and end up in the hospital. She was in and out of intensive care frequently.

A year after his death, I was already practicing magnetic therapy on myself using all the equipment my father had left behind. That same year, while still studying in New York, I was in a car accident that left me with severe whiplash. I healed from the pain and trauma using magnetic therapy on myself and chiropractic adjustments I received at a clinic in Forest Hills.

At that clinic, I did an externship, similar to an internship, but shorter, offered through the university. There, I learned about applied kinesiology, which helped me understand how to "diagnose" by testing muscle response through touch and movement. This technique applied not just to vertebral subluxations, but also to determining the polarity a patient might need, based on whether their condition was hyperactive or underactive. The chiropractors I trained under, Dr. José Rodríguez and his associate, not only treated my neck. They taught me a great deal.

I completed my main internship at the chiropractic college clinic on the Glen Cove campus. I was one of the few students who completed all required hours and still chose to go to another clinic on Fridays and Saturdays to keep learning.

Even though I was feeling better, I still suffered from migraines. So my mom flew in and brought me more magnets to treat the headaches during my final exams. I recovered and passed all my tests!

When I finished my internship and returned to Puerto Rico, I opened a small clinic in the same space where my father once had his. I started with half of my mom's terrace and ended up taking over the whole thing. I expanded from three treatment rooms to eight. (Yes, I paid rent!) My mom helped apply magnetic therapy to patients, which kept her busy and distracted until she started talking about my dad again.

I would have loved the opportunity to work alongside my father, to continue learning directly from him. But as I began seeing patients and providing treatment, I realized that my personal experiences had given me a unique perspective. My life's journey has deeply enriched my career because no one understands a patient quite like someone who has been one. I have been both a patient and a lifelong apprentice of this field, and for that, I am profoundly grateful.

As my practice grew, the media began taking notice, and I started receiving interview requests about chiropractic care and the benefits of magnetic therapy. I became an advocate for these treatments, sharing their advantages across various platforms: radio, television, and print. After all, I was the first, and at the time only, female Puerto Rican chiropractor. I also gave talks and lectures at institutions like Puerto Rico Junior College, Ana G. Méndez University System, Interamerican University, and more. I wanted to spread the word about the incredible benefits of properly practiced magnetic therapy, just like my father once had.

I met my husband when I was eight years old. As I mentioned earlier, he lived just two doors down from us. Although we had known each other since childhood, it wasn't until the summer of 1982, the summer before my father passed away, that we formed an immediate and lasting connection. That bond remains strong to this day. He has always been my right hand, my greatest supporter.

When I started my practice in Puerto Rico, he put his knowledge of electronics to use, wiring the entire office. He installed electrical outlets and fans to keep patients comfortable while they waited, among many other improvements.

Our marriage has always been filled with happiness and mutual respect. Our family grew quickly, and within five years, we had three children: Jorge Rafael, Adrián José, and Alexandra Cecilia.

My husband eagerly accompanied me to conventions and seminars. Eventually, he became involved in the practice itself, assisting with magnetic therapy sessions. He was so inspired by the work that he took a course to become a chiropractic assistant. I loved seeing how passionate he became about what we were doing. With each trip, his interest and love for the field grew. It didn't take much to convince him to study chiropractics. Once he completed his prerequisites, he went to finish his degree in Georgia, when I was expecting our youngest, Alexandra.

While my husband was in the United States studying, I remained in Puerto Rico with our three children. During that time, I accepted a research fellowship focused on pediatric chiropractic care through the International Chiropractic Pediatric Association with Dr. Larry Webster. Webster is best known for developing the Webster Technique, a method that helps position breech babies correctly during pregnancy. The fellowship consisted of ten courses, each lasting twelve hours, over the span of eight weeks. Since my studies required travel, I took every opportunity to visit my husband, often bringing Alexandra with me. Our children have always been our priority, and these visits allowed him to stay connected to her development. Jorge and Adrián would join us whenever they were on school break.

I became certified in the Webster Technique, once again becoming the first Puerto Rican woman with a title. Today, my daughter, Alexandra, also practices this technique, and she loves her craft.

Some time later, I began developing carpal tunnel syndrome due to improper positioning during the countless chiropractic adjustments I had performed throughout my career. I started treating my wrists with magnets at home, but I knew I was facing a serious challenge. This injury would take time to heal, and if I wasn't careful, it could impact the quality of care I provided to my patients.

Around this time, while attending a chiropractic convention, I noticed wrist support bands being sold at a store. Seeing them sparked an idea: what if I combined the support pads with properly positioned magnets to provide continuous treatment and even aid in long-term recovery? I decided to test my theory by modifying a band with the same magnet I had been using to treat my wrist pain. I wore it all day, and to my delight, it was a complete success. I called this magnet the *domino* due to its size, measuring one inch by two inches.

By applying the magnetic field daily and receiving chiropractic adjustments to the affected joint, I was able to continue working pain-free.

This breakthrough led to another idea: why not develop similar magnetic devices for other types of treatment? My father, Ralph U. Sierra, had also experimented with this approach in his practice. He designed different bands for various parts of the body, and they were so effective that Dr. Barton W. DuKett once wrote an article titled *The Magic Bands of Dr. Sierra* in reference to their success. The field of biomagnetism was evolving, and by then, the market already offered magnetic support products with built-in magnets.

> These bands became both my inspiration and a resource to create devices for patients to continue their treatment at home. Among the equipment I inherited from my father, I found his magnetizing machine, and the rest is history.

In the beginning, my mother helped in making the bands. As demand grew, we trained assistants who took over production. *Sierra's Magnetic Bands* needed a secure fastening system to ensure proper placement on the body. I began researching these accessories to better understand their functionality and, most importantly, to verify whether they were using the correct polarity: the negative north pole facing the body. I also examined the strength of the magnets and their gauss levels, as these factors were essential in determining the depth of penetration and effectiveness in treating affected areas.

As I began experimenting with magnetic bands, I ordered products from Asia and Canada to test their effectiveness. I still have boxes filled with incorrect magnets and poor imitations. That's why, when we first started producing our own magnetic bands, we made it a priority to ensure that the therapeutic side, the negative north pole, was properly identified and positioned for the best results. We carefully selected high-quality magnets and meticulously evaluated every magnetic accessory before incorporating it into our designs.

In the past, since my father handcrafted these bands himself, we called them *Sierra's Originals*. Over the years, I refined the design and modified some of the original specifications to enhance their effectiveness. Today, these bands are part of my *Dr. Sierra Magnet Collection*.

With time, I found a factory capable of manufacturing jewelry, tubes, and braces for the knees, elbows, hands, and ankles, each embedded with appropriately placed magnets of the correct strength. These new designs were just as powerful as *Sierra's Originals*. I also expanded the product line, creating magnetic face and eye masks, and even a magnetic hairbrush.

Throughout my life, magnetic therapy has repeatedly helped me recover from conditions and complications brought on by conventional medicine. All three of my children were born via C-section. In each case, I had to accept general anesthesia because I was unwilling to allow needles near my spinal cord. The physical toll of anesthesia, combined with the invasiveness of the surgical procedure, was significant. However, once again, magnetic therapy played a key role in my rapid and full recovery.

Magnetic therapy was also instrumental in helping me heal from a skiing accident. I injured my knee so severely that doctors recommended arthroscopic surgery. From the day of the injury, I wore a magnetic tube wrap on my knee consistently. My recovery was so remarkable that my orthopedic doctor is still waiting for me to schedule the procedure! Within three months, my knee had significantly improved. I am 100% certain this was thanks to my consistent use of magnetic therapy.

Once my husband finished his degree and returned to Puerto Rico, we moved our clinic to a more commercial location. Now there were two chiropractors in the office! I initially thought this transition would give me more time with our three children, but in reality, I ended up blending my work and family life even more. While managing the clinic I also kept my kids active, enrolling them in martial arts, dance, and various sports. It was a fantastic time: busy, exhausting, but deeply rewarding and special.

However, as life often reminds us, we can't do it all. My schedule became so packed that I didn't have the time to continue my father's studies and research into the magnetic field. My greatest aspiration was to expand knowledge in this area, reaching more patients and providing relief to as many people as possible.

Although my schedule was always full, I loved being with my patients and witnessing their gradual improvements. I also cherished being a mother, and watching my children grow up was a joy. However, no matter how much I loved it all, the daily rush often leads us to neglect ourselves. My time was more limited than before, but I still made sure to stay active and keep moving. I am always learning and evolving.

At our office, the *Jarrot Sierra Clinic*, we turned a dream into reality. I was able to establish my own practice and, although I never had the chance to work alongside my father, I opened the clinic with someone who valued it just as much as he would have. On the clinic's TVs, we play educational presentations, as well as photos and videos of Sierra. My father's legacy is woven into everything.

Among the many things my father taught us, one of the most valuable was to pay attention to our dreams. After opening the clinic, I had a dream in which I was guided to modify the magnetic therapy process. With our understanding that the negative north pole energy is beneficial, while the positive south pole energy can stimulate and accelerate the development of illnesses, my husband and I began to innovate.

We designed a magnetic table equipped with copper coils and magnets, ensuring that all the negative north pole energy reached the patient while redirecting the positive south pole energy downward, preventing any potential harm. I firmly believe that my father's condition deteriorated due to his prolonged exposure to the positive south pole energy. At the time, the practice of biomagnetism was still in its early stages and had not yet been refined. I am certain he would be proud of our achievement, knowing that today, both chiropractors and patients can benefit safely from magnetic therapy.

In 1998, I served as vice president of the Puerto Rico Chiropractic Association, and later, I was elected president. In 2001, Governor Sila María Calderón appointed me to the Puerto Rico Board of Chiropractic Examiners, the very board my father founded in 1952. When Governor Aníbal Acevedo Vilá took office, he reappointed me as president. The board consists of three members, all appointed by the governor, and is responsible for ensuring that chiropractors adhere to the law and meet the necessary qualifications to practice in Puerto Rico. I held this position for seven years and loved every aspect of my work.

By 2004, I decided to formally launch my line of magnetic therapy products. That year, we opened *Health Magnetic Store & More*, which remains active in the market today. We loved the store's location so much that we eventually relocated the clinic right next door. That same year, my eldest son left for the United States to study chiropractic care. During this period of growth and expansion, while focusing on our children's education and forging new paths, my mother passed away. She was a woman of immense love, dedication, and strong values. She maintained her health with chiropractic adjustments and magnetic therapy until the very end. I will always carry with me the love she had for her family and her legacy of self-care.

Our children followed in our footsteps. All three of them became chiropractors. It fills me with immense joy and pride!

As for the clinic, over time, I became increasingly frustrated. **I was tired of medical insurance companies and health plans pretending to know more about chiropractic care than those who dedicated their entire life to the profession.** After twenty-five years of practice, I had had enough of battling bureaucracy and nonsensical processes. I decided to leave the clinic and focus solely on the store and my research into biomagnetism. What I didn't anticipate were the financial challenges this transition would bring, compounded by the economic recession that affected both the USA and Puerto Rico.

The change in my work routine hit me hard. I went from being active all day, on my feet, engaging with patients, building connections, and sharing laughter, to sitting in an office, buried in administration, computers, and endless paperwork. The more time passed, the more I felt lost in this new role. But at least I was still researching, developing new health and magnetic therapy products, and working with magnets and supplements!

Then, one day at the office, a box fell onto my head. I treated the injury with magnets and it improved. But, about three weeks later, the day before an upcoming trip, my shoulder froze in place. My son Jorge was already practicing, and he treated me with a brief session of laser therapy.

Speaking of laser therapy, cold laser therapy is a form of phototherapy, or light therapy. This technique uses a red light beam that, when applied to an injured area, stimulates the healing process. When the tissue absorbs the light, biological reactions occur at the cellular level, making this therapy particularly effective for acute injuries. The combination of laser therapy and biomagnetic principles further accelerates recovery. My father, when drafting the chiropractic law in 1952, included light therapy as an approved modality. This means that, by law, every chiropractor in Puerto Rico can offer this treatment in their offices.

When I boarded the plane for my trip, my hands swelled up. The cold weather left me almost completely incapacitated. Even so, the adjustments my husband performed and the magnets I used made the trip bearable. Upon returning to Puerto Rico, I decided to undergo lab tests to determine if something was affecting me beyond what I could see at a glance. The results confirmed that I had rheumatoid arthritis.

That same year, I attended a chiropractic seminar where JJ Virgin was a guest speaker, promoting her book *The Seven Foods to Avoid and How to Lose Seven Pounds in Seven Days*. I had gained some weight, so I decided to adjust my diet. By returning to the foods I knew were beneficial for me and eliminating others, I gradually regained my routine and reconnected with my healthier lifestyle.

Over time, along with my new eating habits, I started feeling better. However, the rheumatoid nodules kept reappearing. My doctor, a chiropractor specializing in nutrition, determined that the underlying cause was stress. His consistent recommendation was for me to take time off work, but at that moment, that simply wasn't an option.

Before transitioning to administrative work, I had been completely pain-free. I had excellent lab results, practiced yoga daily, stretched regularly, and had full mobility to bend, move, and work with ease. I couldn't comprehend how stress could be responsible for all the discomfort I was experiencing. Of course, we all go through stressful situations, but in my case, they had never lasted long. The administrative workload was heavy, but I balanced it with all the wellness routines and techniques I had developed over the years.

I wore my magnetic jewelry daily while working, took my supplements correctly, and maintained a well-balanced diet. I placed a magnet on my desk chair to sit on, kept two magnets on the floor to rest my feet, and at night, I wore magnetic bands and supports. I did everything I knew was best for me.

I have always loved my profession and felt grateful to work in a field I am deeply passionate about. So, I struggled to understand how my doctor could insist that stress was affecting me and suggest that I take a break from the very thing I loved most.

This situation made me take a step back and reflect on my life. I began prioritizing myself, truly enjoying each moment, and allowing things to flow instead of constantly worrying. In this process of introspection, I started questioning what stress really was. That's when I finally uncovered the root of my problem.

When the body is under stress, it instinctively activates the *fight or flight* response as a survival mechanism, sensing a potential threat. This triggers a surge of adrenaline and cortisol, preparing the body to either flee or defend itself. During this process, the body falls out of equilibrium (homeostasis). Normally, once the perceived threat is gone, the body regains balance. However, as the saying goes, *no ailment lasts a century, and none could endure such,* but the body also cannot withstand a prolonged state of alertness and emergency. And there it was, my answer!

Even though I didn't feel stress, I was carrying a significant burden of it. Finally understanding this allowed me to establish a new sense of balance. I went through an adaptation process that made me more aware of what my body was going through. That's why it's important not to get used to imbalance. Once it becomes the norm, we don't recognize it as a problem until the body eventually implodes.

Focusing on restoring my energy was essential to over-coming this temporary survival mode. I became increasingly curious about the body's energy, that natural electrical charge we all possess. I began exploring quantum physics, looking into the invisible field of light and information that surrounds us.

I came to understand that as my stress hormones increased, my invisible energy fields, both internal and external, diminished, even when I felt physically energetic. This realization led me back to my father's teachings and his fundamental principle: *we are energy.*

I reconnected with the knowledge of our aura, chakras, and the magnetic fields that surround us. Every living being possesses these elements. Even plants have an aura. If neglected, this invisible field of light that fills our chakras and aura continuously weakens.

My condition reignited my studies in electromagnetic therapy. During this period, I discovered a wealth of literature on Pulsed Electromagnetic Field Therapy (PEMF), and I was amazed by the extensive research and published studies that confirmed the benefits of magnetic therapy.

It was no longer just my father's word and mine against the world, there was scientific validation. I obtained state-of-the-art equipment from Germany, Switzerland, Canada, and Hungary to further explore its applications.

PEMF is used to improve circulation and enhance cellular metabolism. Later in this book, you will find an entire chapter dedicated to this topic. Today, there are methods and studies on PEMF from six different scientists, including Sierra. Understanding these approaches is essential for recharging cells and offering effective therapeutic healing to patients.

My research also led me to make adjustments in my own routine and the way I conducted therapy sessions. Now, I incorporate PEMF therapy multiple times a day for thirty to forty minutes, even while traveling.

The key for me has been to use full-body PEMF equipment, as well as chair-sized and half-back devices. I also reintegrated daily meditation into my routine, just as I did when I was younger. Staying active became a priority again, and I primarily practice Qi Gong. Whenever possible, I walk, even on the beach.

I ensure I get enough rest, eat nutrient-rich foods, and keep my heart filled with gratitude and joy. This holistic approach helped me recover my energy and reignite my passion for learning and creating. The book you now hold in your hands exists because of this transformation, because of the life changes and self-care practices that restored my well-being.

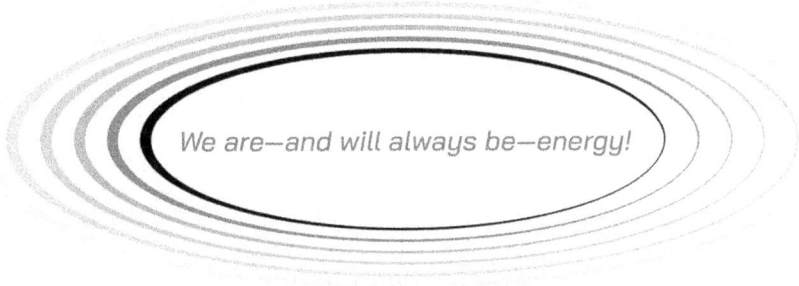

We are—and will always be—energy!

Sierra and Davis' Story

D
r. Ralph U. Sierra was an alumnus of Albert Roy Davis in 1967. His connection with Davis deepened when he was diagnosed with Ménière's disease, followed by prostate inflammation, for which he refused surgery. Davis helped him restore his health through science and biomagnetism therapy, which gained recognition in both Puerto Rico and the United States. His case contributed to its gradual integration into medical practices and chiropractic offices, broadening its acceptance.

This chapter explores the relationship between two visionary minds, their correspondence, and their shared understanding of biomagnetism, its science, and its transformative effects on the human body.

Their Lives

Meet Ralph U. Sierra

D
r. Ralph U. Sierra was born on December 6, 1904, in San Juan, Puerto Rico. Deeply fascinated by human biology and the potential of the human body, he earned a degree in minor surgery in 1922 and, in 1924, moved to Brooklyn, New York, to further his studies. In 1927, he graduated from the Chicago Engineering Institute as an Applied Electrical Engineer and later obtained a bachelor's degree from Virginia Eastern College. When the Great Depression hit and he lost his job, Dr. Sierra shifted his focus to physical therapy. In 1932, he studied massage and physical therapy at the Chicago National College. Afterwards, he returned to New York, where he worked as a physical therapist at Bellevue and Kings County Hospital for over fourteen years. Later, he studied chiropractic care at Atlantic States, which led him to an instructor position at the Columbia Institute of

Chiropractic in New York. Eventually, he became a licensed chiropractor in Nevada, Wyoming, Maryland, and Puerto Rico.

In 1948, Dr. Sierra introduced chiropractic care to Puerto Rico, where it was officially recognized as a legal practice in 1952. He was the first person ever to receive a chiropractic license on the island.

He was also instrumental in creating the legislation that established the *Junta Examinadora de Quiroprácticos* (Puerto Rico Board of Chiropractic Examiners), ensuring that chiropractors in Puerto Rico could obtain official licenses to practice.

Dr. Sierra was deeply involved in research on tuberculosis, poliomyelitis (polio), and childhood paralysis. He officially opened his chiropractic practice in 1950 and was also recognized as a nutritionist and sports medicine specialist.

He served as president of the *Hospital Pediátrico de Niños Mentalmente Incapacitados* (Pediatric Hospital for Mentally Handicapped Children) and was an active member of the 32nd Degree Mason Shriners Club, Lions Club, Master Key, and Elks. Additionally, he was the Caribbean director for Miss World Queen of Posture & Physical Fitness, a spiritual minister, and the author of three books. He was also a distinguished member of the American Association for the Advancement of Science and the United Federation of Science, and he was accepted into the New York Academy of Sciences, a momentous achievement, evidenced by his preserved acceptance letter.

Throughout his career, Dr. Sierra gave hundreds of lectures across the United States, Canada, Central America, and the Caribbean. Scientists from Japan, Russia, India, France, Canada, South America, and the USA, visited his laboratory, corresponded with him, and sought his insights. His letters and records include addresses from places as diverse as Trinidad & Tobago, Denmark, South Africa, England, the Philippines, Nepal, Venezuela, Colombia, and Quebec, Canada, where he also delivered a lecture.

In 1964, he began to suffer debilitating dizziness, which impacted his ability to practice. Despite consulting multiple specialists in the USA and Puerto Rico, no one could diagnose the cause of his condition.

Meet Albert Roy Davis

Albert Roy Davis, Ph.D., was a pioneering scientist and investigator born in Halifax, Nova Scotia. In 1936, he founded the Albert Roy Davis Research Laboratory in Green Cove Springs, Florida, dedicated to studying the magnetic effects on both organic and inorganic systems. His work led to discovering the existence of two distinct energies within magnetism.

In 1959, Davis introduced the science of biomagnetism and its applications to control and alleviate diseases in India. He played a crucial role in the education and development of doctors and scientists in West Bengal, India, including Dr. A. K. Bhattacharya, D.C., Ph.D. That's why, in 1967, Bhattacharya referred Sierra to Davis, recognizing that Florida was much closer to Puerto Rico than India. This introduction sparked a collaboration that would propel the field of biomagnetism into global recognition.

While studying at the University of Florida in 1936, Davis observed that the north (negative) and south (positive) poles of a magnet produced different effects when applied to biological systems. Not only did he confirm the health benefits of magnets, but he also recognized that Earth itself functions as a giant magnet, divided into north and south poles, each influencing both living organisms and inert matter differently (*The Magnetic Blueprint of Life*, Davis, n.d.).

Through his discoveries, Davis found that magnets could be used to minimize and eliminate cancerous cells in animals, as well as treat conditions such as arthritis, glaucoma, infertility, and other illnesses associated with aging. **His research led him to conclude that the negative north pole of a magnet has beneficial and healing effects, while the positive south pole exerts a stressful influence on biological systems.**

Sierra & Davis' Collaboration

In 1960, at the suggestion of Dr. A. K. Bhattacharyya, Dr. Ralph U. Sierra began corresponding with Albert Roy Davis. Eager to explore the potential of biomagnetism, Sierra actively participated in Davis's research—not only seeking relief for his own ailments but also contributing to Davis's ongoing discoveries.

After experiencing firsthand the remarkable benefits of biomagnetism and magnetic therapy, Sierra introduced the practice to Puerto Rico in 1967. Just two years later, in 1969, he established the Puerto Rico Scientific Research Laboratory, where he continued his collaboration with Davis. As Sierra deepened his expertise in biomagnetism, he dedicated himself to educating others, delivering lectures on the use of magnets to improve health.

Thanks to his efforts, thousands of people across Puerto Rico, the United States, Mexico, Canada, Spain, India, and South America benefited from this knowledge. Dr. Sierra played an active role in clinical research on biomagnetism and helped expand awareness of magnetic energy throughout North and South America from the late 1970s into the early 1980s. During this time, he compiled an extensive collection of data on the therapeutic use of negative magnetic fields, particularly in treating arthritis, musculoskeletal disorders, and cancer patients.

His work led to the development of specialized magnetic bands for the neck, knees, and back, as well as the creation of his own mechanical coil, an innovation that would later evolve into a recognized form of magnetic therapy. With this technology, he and his team designed the *inverted electromagnetic table*, which featured positive south poles directed toward the floor.

Thousands of people experienced the benefits of biomagnetic therapy, including numerous professional athletes who found relief through Sierra's treatments. His expertise culminated in the publication of two essential works: *Energía magnética o biomagnetismo* (Magnetic Energy or Biomagnetism) and *Power in a Magnet*, both of which continue to serve as valuable sources of information on the subject.

One day, at seventy-five years old, Dr. Sierra climbed a mango tree to magnetize it by hammering in a steel nail. After completing the task, as he began to climb down, he slipped and fell hard on his back. Although he did not suffer any fractures, the fall triggered a resurgence of the prostate condition that had disappeared for over fifteen years.

Compounding the issue, Dr. Sierra had been constantly exposed to the South pole positive energy while administering therapy to his patients. This side of the magnetic field, as we know, stimulates growth and propagation, including that of undesirable conditions.

Even while unwell, Dr. Sierra continued treating patients and traveling to give lectures throughout South America, the Dominican Republic, and the United States. (A curious detail: the mango tree he magnetized bore hundreds of sweet mangos.)

Though Albert Roy Davis is rightly recognized as the father of modern biomagnetism, Dr. Ralph U. Sierra devoted his life to the science as well. He helped spread the word, experimented boldly, deepened our understanding of magnetic polarities, and developed tools and protocols that made this therapy accessible. Over time, these methods have been refined so that we may fully harness the healing potential of this incredible science.

Discoveries

(This section is written from Dr. Ralph U. Sierra's point of view.)

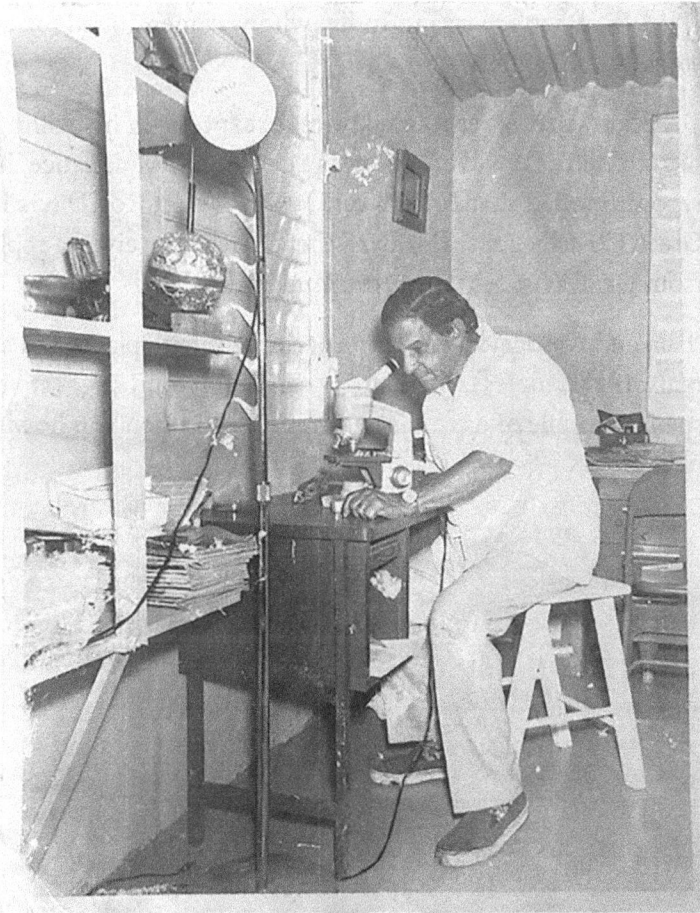

My condition [vertigo] worsened by the day. No medical treatment could provide relief. After consulting nearly every otorhinolaryngologist both locally and abroad, I sought help from osteopaths, chiropractors, and even a psychic healer, but all in vain. My condition deteriorated to the point that I once pleaded with a neurosurgeon friend to inject me with anything, to do anything he could to my vestibular nerve. When he refused, I realized I would have to endure this suffering on my own.

In 1967, I came across an article written by Joseph Goodavage in *Fate* magazine titled *Man, the Biomagnetic Animal.* The article left a profound impression on me, and I immediately wrote to Dr. A. K. Bhattacharya in India, who was mentioned for his work with magnets.

Dr. Bhattacharya responded by mail, expressing his willingness to help. However, given the geographical distance, he recommended that I reach out to Dr. Albert Roy Davis in Green Cove Springs, Florida. When I finally received a reply from Dr. Davis, his words intrigued me.

"I am an investigator, and my experience is with plants and animals. Nevertheless, I am sure I can help you. I suggest you spend a couple of days here with me. I can teach you how to help others."

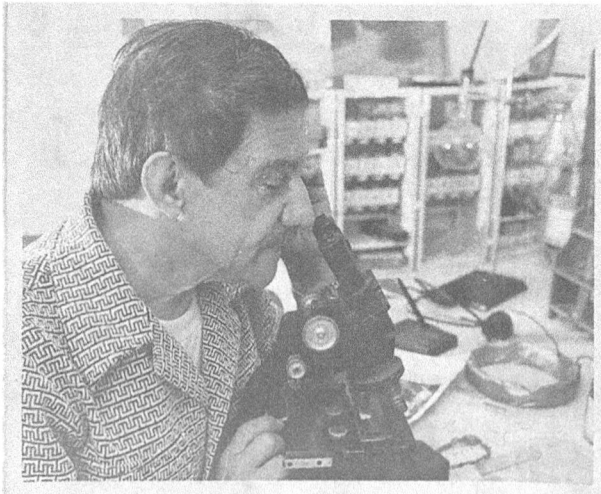

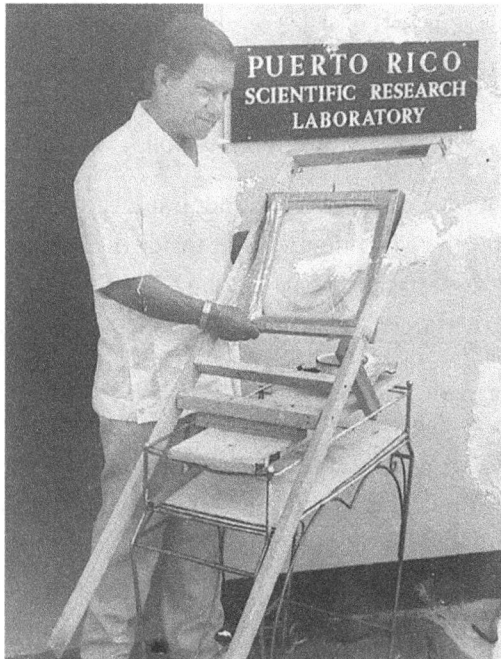

At that time, I was experiencing one of the worst health crises of my life. The vertigo episodes were relentless, and I often felt a numbing sensation in my head and neck. I was afraid to travel alone, so I invited a fellow doctor, Dr. Avilés, who was also interested in the field, to accompany me. We arrived in Green Cove early in the morning. Dr. Davis suggested we check into our hotel first, but I insisted.

"Let Dr. Avilés handle that while you see what you can do for me. I feel extremely dizzy."

"Come in," he said.

He took samples of my saliva and urine before remarking, *"Man, you're full of acid."* He then placed a magnetic earphone in my ear and showed me a small magnetic stick. Dropping it into a cup of water mixed with a teaspoon of baking soda, he stirred the liquid counterclockwise.

"Magnetic energy from the north moves to the left," he explained.

At that moment, his words sounded like pure nonsense. My only thought was, *My God, I traveled all this way just to listen to a mad scientist. After seeing so many esteemed doctors, how could this man possibly help me with such a foolish theory?*

Yet, I followed his instructions and drank the mixture. The earphone produced strange sounds inside my middle ear, which I had never experienced before. Believe it or not, by the time Dr. Avilés returned from the hotel, my head felt significantly better.

That marked the beginning of our learning journey. Dr. Avilés, with master's degrees and a Ph.D. in electronics and electrical engineering, grasped the concepts more quickly than I did. Roy, as I now call him, was a natural teacher. His laboratory was a gathering place for scientists and professors from various universities. The five days I spent there changed my life.

We learned truths that are often misrepresented in many institutions and universities. I was amazed at how he measured a magnet's potency, identified the correct polarity, and, most importantly, demonstrated that a magnet has not just two poles but a third, neutral side. He emphasized that magnetism consists of two distinct energies, contradicting the common belief that it is a homogeneous force. He showed us firsthand how these energies affect biological systems.

We covered an entire year's worth of college-level study in just one week. By then, I was even able to eat apple pie, one of the foods that had previously triggered my worst vertigo episodes.

I returned home filled with enthusiasm, carrying new books, notes, six magnetic cylinders for polarizing water, and two magnetic plates, one measuring 2" x 6" and the other 2" x 3". This marked the beginning of my own laboratory.

A friend, who was also a doctor, had two elderly white rats that he planned to dispose of before they died. I saw an opportunity to experiment. I applied both north and south poles outside their cage. Within a week, they were remarkably rejuvenated. I could hardly believe they were the same rats my friend had given me. Initially, I had used two horseshoe magnets facing each other, with one side north and the other south.

Curious about these results, I purchased some mice. I applied the north pole to one group, the south pole to another, and left the third group as a control, without any magnetic exposure. The results were striking: The rats exposed to the north pole became lean and energetic, but the ones under the south pole grew sluggish and overweight.

One day, I placed the magnets too close to the rats, and they all appeared to fall asleep. At first, I thought they were hypnotized. I removed them from the cages except for one, which remained exposed to the south pole's magnetic field. To my shock, it died.

To confirm my findings, I repeated the experiment. Again, the rat exposed to strong south pole energy perished in under thirty minutes. This led me to a crucial realization: **prolonged exposure to a strong south magnetic field is dangerous.** From that point forward, I knew I had to be extremely cautious when using south pole energy.

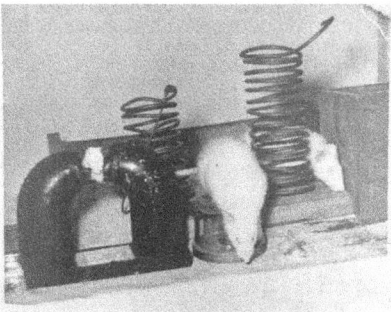

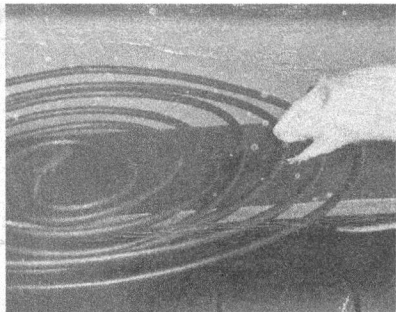

Six months later, I returned to Green Cove Springs, where I found myself surrounded by scientists, doctors, engineers, and a distinguished oceanographer. We exchanged ideas and shared our research findings. They seemed to be impressed with my experiments, and while we were all present, Dr. Davis confirmed the fatal effects of prolonged exposure to the south magnetic field in rats.

A representative from the Florida Department of Agriculture was also in attendance and provided insights on the effects of polarized water on soil that Davis watered using magnetically treated water once or twice a day. Here was a significant increase in calcium, magnesium, and other essential nutrients.

When I returned home after my second visit, I started my own magnetic garden. At the same time, I began treating patients suffering from arthritis, bursitis, rheumatoid conditions, and various neurological disorders. Many showed gradual improvement, but the biggest challenge was convincing patients to continue treatment at home. Despite this, I was not discouraged, as those who believed the benefits of biomagnetism followed my instructions and achieved remarkable levels of healing.

In 1969, I attended a conference in San Diego, California. At that time, I didn't have many cases to report, but soon after, someone published an article about a case study I had shared, about a woman suffering from uterine cancer who had severe vaginal bleeding. Thanks to magnetic treatments, her bleeding stopped, and she was even able to return to work.

Suddenly, I began receiving letters from all over the world, like Germany, Hungary, England, Canada, Australia, and beyond, all asking for advice. However, the highlight of this experience was a visit from Dr. Kenneth McLean, a gynecologist and cancer specialist also mentioned in the article.

Dr. McLean initially planned to stay for three days, but he ended up extending his visit to a full week. We discussed magnetism, and during one of our conversations, he famously stated: "Cancer cannot exist within a high magnetic field." Upon returning to New York, he installed a laboratory in his office, where he personally validated the truth of his statement over and over again.

Then came 1972, a defining year for the Puerto Rico Scientific Research Laboratory. It was during this time that we hosted Dr. Justa Smith, along with a biologist and a team of Japanese scientists, all eager to observe our laboratory and magnetic garden.

These were highly regarded scientists who already understood the value of magnetic energy. Dr. Justa Smith, a Ph.D. in philosophy from New York, had demonstrated through her research that strong magnetic fields affect the reactivity of specific enzymes within the human body (Cook & Smith, 1964). The Japanese delegation was particularly fascinating. It included two doctors, two engineers, a physicist, a biologist and an interpreter. Among them was Dr. Kyoki Nakagawa, who, in 1976, would go on to present a thesis at the *Third Conference on Magnetic Fields and Living Bodies* in Tokyo, titled *The Magnetic Field Deficiency Syndrome* (Nakagawa, 1976). The Japanese research on this topic had actually begun as early as 1958.

1970 – Water & Magnets

(The words of Dr. Sierra as he wrote them.)

Liver fibrosis occurs when the liver undergoes repeated damage. After an injury, even a severe one like acute hepatitis, the liver generally repairs itself by creating new liver cells and integrating them into the network of internal connective tissue left behind when previous liver cells die. However, when the damage is repetitive or chronic, such as in cases of chronic hepatitis, the liver continuously attempts to repair itself, leading to the formation of scar tissue, also known as fibrosis. The progression of fibrosis accelerates when the underlying cause is a bile duct obstruction, which can also result in a yellowish discoloration of the skin.

I have observed that suspending a 300-gauss magnet with a 5/8-inch diameter and a length of ½ to ¾ inches in water for one minute gradually dissolves flaky calcium deposits. A similar effect is achieved using a cylindrical magnet measuring 5/8-inch in diameter and 3 inches in length, with a strength of 1,000 gauss, when suspended in a 16-ounce cup of water for one minute and consumed twice daily.

It appears that this method may also help reduce the hardening or fibrosis of the liver.

(End of Dr. Sierra's excerpt.)

The Figure Eight

The figure eight represents the union of positive and negative energies in nature. It is such a fundamental and recurring pattern that even DNA and RNA, the very structures that form the basis of life, take on a shape reminiscent of an eight. In nature, positive energy spins to the right, while negative energy spins to the left. These energies are in constant motion, never static, continuously interacting and combining. For that reason, it is essential to use each type of energy appropriately in order to achieve the desired outcomes. Magnetism and electricity are inseparable; they always coexist.

The magnetic field of the negative north pole moves in a counterclockwise direction, while the positive south pole moves clockwise. This type of energetic movement, often referred to as a vortex, is commonly discussed in scientific literature. However, one important fact is often overlooked: it was Albert Roy Davis who first discovered this phenomenon, and Dr. Ralph U. Sierra who later confirmed it. Although both Davis and Sierra are credited with a chapter in the history of the electrovibrating body, many contributors to this field have yet to receive the recognition they deserve from the broader scientific community.

Davis was the first to observe that magnetism flows within and around a magnet in a figure-eight shape. He challenged the method introduced by Michael Faraday in 1852 to illustrate the "lines of force" around a magnet. Faraday's method involved placing iron shavings on a sheet of flat paper and then positioning a magnet underneath. However, this method presents a misconception. When iron shavings are placed within a magnetic field, they become temporarily magnetized, essentially turning into small magnets themselves. These particles then attract and repel one another, producing a pattern that misrepresents the true behavior of magnetic energy.

Dr. Sierra proposed a much simpler and more accurate way to visualize these magnetic power lines, a method that can easily be performed in a classroom. The experiment uses a clear glass container filled with cold water and barium ferrite (BaFe), a powdered magnetic material.

Here is the step-by-step technique: Use a transparent glass container, large enough to observe movement clearly, and fill it with cold water. Add ferrite powder, also known as barium ferrite, to the water. Using a cylindrical magnet or a long magnetic bar attached to a non-magnetic handle, stir the water vigorously so the ferrite particles are suspended. Once the particles are thoroughly mixed, stop stirring and hold the magnet vertically at the center of the container. As the water stills, the suspended ferrite particles will gradually align themselves according to the magnetic field, forming a clear figure-eight shape: a visual demonstration of the magnetic energy pattern.

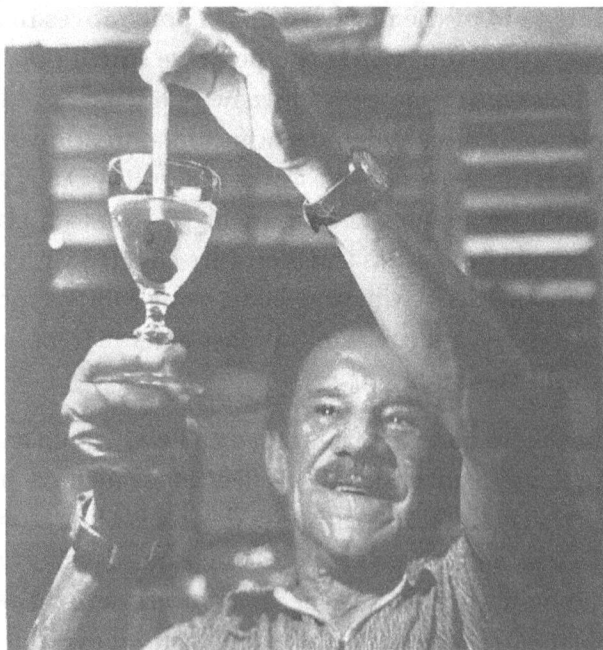

Letters

These are fragments and excerpts from some of the letters written by Dr. Ralph U. Sierra, of which I, his daughter, am the custodian.

July 3rd, 1970

Davis' Comments to the Associated Press

"The Associated Press asked me to provide background on my investigation into biomagnetism. Your name was the first I mentioned as an outstanding scientist who has contributed greatly to proving, through your work, that this science has so much to offer humanity. The story should be featured in every major newspaper. In fact, go look for it. You deserve to be recognized for all your invaluable work and support. I also briefly mentioned Dr. Bhattacharya's contributions in India."

November 13th, 1970

Letter Regarding Tests with Mice

"You are correct in your tests with rats. You must include a group exposed to the [negative] north pole, a group exposed to the [positive] south pole, a control group with no exposure, and a group exposed to the horseshoe magnet (dual polarity). This will undoubtedly reveal behavioral differences similar to those observed in humans depending on whether they were born and raised south or north of the magnetic equator. They will behave much like the people native to those respective geographic regions.

Mothers who give birth in the [positive] south pole don't experience much pain before labor. Mothers who give birth in the [negative] north pole tend to be very sensitive to sound and light, and go through significant pain before and during childbirth.

I covered this thoroughly in the first manuscript I wrote on biomagnetism, which you already have. Read again the section about the baby chicks, on how, while still damp from hatching, they gravitate toward the horseshoe magnet for extended periods, as though seeking the warmth and strength of their mother hen."

May 2nd, 1972

Invitations to assist the conference in November that would take place in Davis' laboratory, sent by Japanese doctors.

May 6th, 1972

Davis mentions his skin disease case and how he managed to control it using magnetic fields.

May 29th, 1972

Kyochi Nakagawa's response, confirming his assistance.

June 5th, 1972

"Magnets, in and of themselves, are not radioactive. However, the energy released by all magnets behaves similarly to a small dose of low-yield cobalt, X-rays, or gamma rays. Davis was working on identifying the exact frequency emitted by our magnets, that is, the frequency of magnetism itself."

October 14th, 1972

"There's nothing we can do during the advanced stages of hepatic insufficiency. However, placing the [negative] north pole (magnet N-1, measuring 2" x 6") over the general liver area for thirty minutes in the morning and again at night has shown results. The kidneys also begin to activate and assist every three days, and I've observed improvement in some cases.

Remember: green, green to yellow, and intense yellow are the stages you can visibly identify by observing the patient's eyes during the investigation. The eyes are crucial, they are the windows of the body and the soul. Always check the eyes."

November 9th, 1972

We know that the [negative] north pole dissolves and draws water into the capillary flow system. This action helps reduce stomach rigidity, which is often caused by gas and by what we call 'cancerous water', the abnormal fluids present in cases of internal cancer.

The water within the subject's body will follow the direction of the north pole when using a 2" x 6" magnet. Always keep this in mind.

Doctors and hospitals often try to insert a long, thick needle into the abdomen to pump out that fluid. This method doesn't work. In fact, in many cases, it can lead to death. Water in those heart cells is under pressure; it cannot simply be pumped out!

September 28th, 1979

"No gallstone tumors. Water polarized with the north pole of the magnet, applied for thirty minutes twice daily, directly over where the gallbladder is located."

December 6th, 1979

"Over the years of investigating the effects of magnetic fields on water, we've consistently proven that when water is treated with the energy of a magnet, whether through AC electromagnets or solid-state permanent magnets, the structure of the water changes. These changes become evident when the treated water is administered to both large and small animals under controlled laboratory conditions.

We have shown that magnetism alters the hardness and soft mineral content of the exposed water. About seven years ago, while you were working with us in the lab, we had a meeting with patent licensing representatives from MIT University. They tested the treated water, and the results confirmed our findings: magnetic fields applied to untreated water currents [...] can remove up to 95% of impurities."

March, 1980

Dr. Ralph U. Sierra traveled to Egypt and measured the pyramid's magnetic strength.

August to September, 1980

Dr. Ralph U. Sierra falls from a treetop.

September 14th, 1980

Sierra Writes to Davis

"I hate to be the bearer of bad news, but they travel fast. I fell from the top of an eight-foot-tall mango tree. The ground was damp and hard, yet I didn't feel any pain at first. The next day, I lifted something heavy and suddenly couldn't stand up straight. I was nearly completely paralyzed.

They took me to the hospital for X-rays. While on the stretcher, they flipped me over. I cried inconsolably from a level of pain I had never known. They laid me in a hospital bed, and I had no energy left. Just a stabbing pain that ran from the top of my head to the soles of my feet. Even my toes hurt.

Back in 1939, when I was diagnosed with prostate cancer, the doctors gave me three years to live. I refused radiation and chemotherapy. My life's work has always warned against them, and accepting those treatments would have discredited everything I've stood for.

Through my travels and lectures around the world, I've shared the science of biomagnetism, this profound, natural, biological, and healing science that drew me into research and sustained me for decades.

I'm now at home, surrounded by my beautiful wife and daughter, who are keeping me well fed and cared for. Please send your prayers and your strength. In this moment of great difficulty, your love and support are more vital than ever.

Your friend always, Ralph."

September 18th, 1980

Davis' Response

"It is with deep sorrow that we received your letter and the news of your fall and resulting paralysis. The first matter to address is how to naturally restore your ability to move and walk.

Based on many similar cases I have investigated here, and with the goal of helping you regain strength and mobility through the results of our biomagnetic research, I offer the following advice:

Please ask Mrs. Sierra and your wonderful, devoted daughter to place two N-1 magnets side by side on the soles of your feet. You'll need four magnets in total. Apply them for forty-five minutes in the morning and again at night. From what I've seen in cases involving falls from ladders, trees, and chairs, general physical strength is often restored within three to four days.

With this method, you'll receive the magnetic fields from both the north and south poles on the lower extremities of your body. I'm also attaching a graphic showing spinal correction and bone fracture support, taken from our most recent research findings.

Please, as soon as your system begins to recover from the shock, let me know how your prostate cancer is progressing. That way, I can update the records and send you the latest findings regarding control through the positive outcomes of our ongoing investigation."

January 6th, 1981

Davis Writes

"I've received a letter and two phone calls about your health and current condition. I've been told that your prostate cancer has progressed, spreading into the lower and now upper regions of your body. I also heard that you've been taking everything available: teas, herbs, tonics, and formulas, in an attempt to reduce the inflammation in your prostate and other affected areas.

Why are you doing this? I know the answer, and so do you. You're clinging so tightly to this mortal illness that you're not thinking clearly anymore.

In the past three years, I've welcomed doctors from numerous international clinics. Together, we've managed to stop prostate cancer. I need you to return to the line of thought, the science you've dedicated yourself to teaching since the day we met.

From the early days of our cancer research, we understood this: cancerous cells are more humid than normal cells, and their membranes contain abnormally high levels of sodium. When we apply the [negative] north pole of the N-1 magnet, we are actively separating these cancerous cells from the excess cancerous water. We are also dissolving the surplus sodium within the cell membranes. Cells that, by their very nature, are trying to shield you from the harmful effects of conventional treatments.

We know the [positive] south pole is a lethal promoter of cancer. Simply being near the surface of the south pole can stimulate the growth and expansion of one or more cancers.

On the other hand, when we place the [negative] north pole of our N-1 magnet over a cancerous area, it draws white blood cells to that region and increases the negative biological voltage of surrounding healthy cells. This inhibits the spread of cancer and starves the cancerous cells already present.

In cases of prostate cancer, we position an N-1 [negative] north pole magnet over a soft-bottomed chair and sit on it for exactly forty-five minutes in the morning and again at night. No more and no less: exactly forty-five minutes.

I ask you, my friend, to have faith. Believe in God. And at the very least, stop and truly consider my suggestions. This could stop your cancer.

I pray to God that you will begin using your magnets on yourself and not only on your patients. You're being exposed to the radiation of the [positive] south pole during your sessions and that is deadly in cases of advanced cancer.

I beg you to remain loyal to our science. Do what we know works. We've seen it stop cancer before. I pray that you do it.

May God guide you and bless you.

Your friend always,

Albert Roy Davis"

November 10th, 1982

Dr. Ralph U. Sierra practiced chiropractic therapy until 1981, and passed away on November 10th, 1982.

The Anatomy of Biomagnetism Book

D r. Ralph U. Sierra is the co-author of the book in which Albert Roy Davis first introduced the concept of biomagnetism to the general public: *The Anatomy of Biomagnetism*. This is clearly stated on the original cover of that publication. However, in a subsequent edition released in 1982 by the publishing house Vantage Press, Dr. Sierra's name was removed from the book entirely.

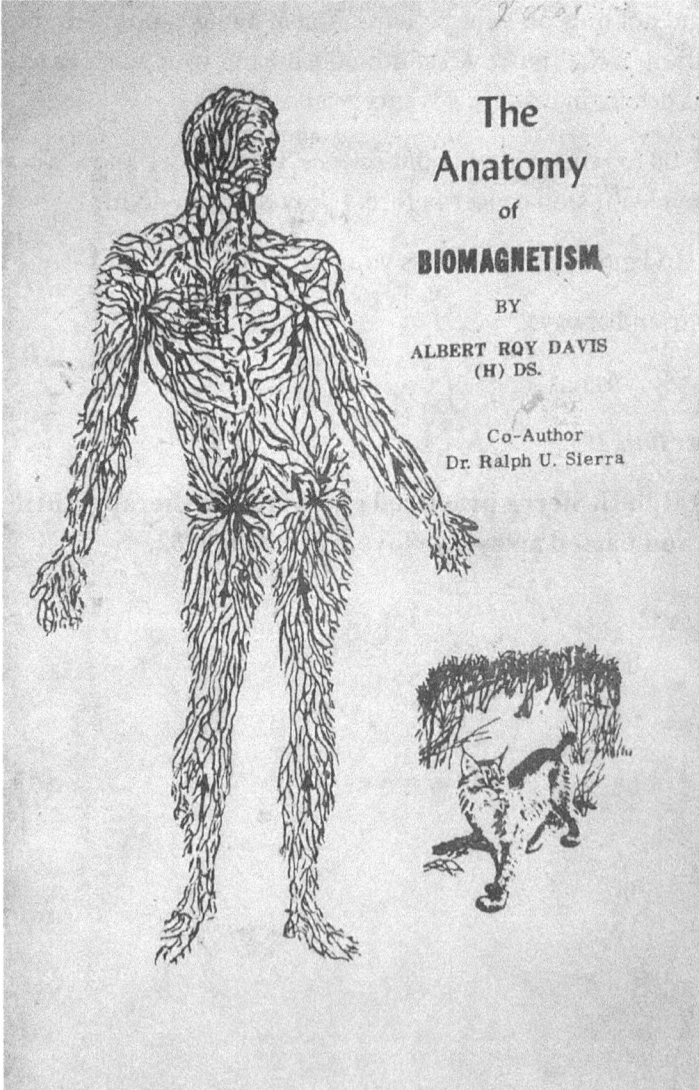

The
Anatomy
of
BIOMAGNETISM
BY
ALBERT ROY DAVIS
(H) DS.

Co-Author
Dr. Ralph U. Sierra

Introduction to Magnetic Fields

Magnetic fields are invisible yet powerful forces that influence electrically charged objects and particles in their surroundings. These fields arise from magnetic activity generated by electrical currents, natural magnets, or magnetized materials. They can exert attractive or repulsive forces on other magnetic objects, and their influence can range from the microscopic to the cosmic scale.

Magnetic fields play a vital role in countless natural processes, from enabling the function of a simple compass to guiding the interaction of subatomic particles. Furthermore, our understanding and manipulation of magnetic fields have led to essential modern technologies, including electronic devices, magnetic resonance imaging (MRI) in medicine, and breakthroughs in numerous scientific disciplines. This fascinating and multifaceted phenomenon continues to be the focus of study and innovation across fields such as physics, medicine, engineering, and space exploration.

What Is a Magnetic Field?

A magnetic field is a manifestation of electromagnetism, one of the four fundamental forces of nature alongside gravity, the strong nuclear force, and the weak nuclear force. This invisible force surrounds both magnets and any object carrying an electric charge in motion. It extends outward from a magnet's negative north pole and inward toward its positive south pole.

When an electric charge moves through a magnetic field, it experiences a perpendicular force relative to its direction of motion. This is known as the magnetic force. This force often causes the charged particle to follow a curved or circular path along the lines of the magnetic field. This principle is closely tied to Faraday's law of induction, which states that the electric voltage induced in a circuit is proportional to the rate of change of the magnetic flux passing through it (Matan, 2023).

Magnetic fields can also be generated by electric currents flowing through a conductor, such as a wire. In such cases, the magnetic field forms concentric rings around the conductor, and the field's strength is directly related to the amount of current that flows through.

The intensity of a magnetic field is measured in Teslas (T) according to the International System of Units (SI). Other commonly used units include the gauss (G) and the oersted (Oe).

We Are Energy

Energy Gives Life to Matter

For as long as I can remember, my father used to say that human beings are energy. When I was younger, I believed he was referring to the invisible magnetic fields emitted by magnets and how they pass through the human body. But as time went on, I came to understand that what he meant was far more spectacular.

Our bodies are made up of atoms. In fact, everything around us is primarily composed of atoms: collections of particles held together by gravitational or chemical forces that give form to everything we see. This means that, since we are made of the same atomic material as the air we breathe, the oceans, and the stars, we all interact with and are affected by the energy that surrounds us, a force that shapes our planet and the entire universe.

Your hand may appear solid, but it is, in reality, a cluster of atoms with space between them, atoms that vibrate within that space. That "empty" space, both within and around the body, is energy. If you were to place your hand under a microscope, you would see a pulsating mass of energy. You share atomic components with the ocean, with celestial bodies, and with the vast universe beyond our comprehension.

How can atoms form everything? Each atom contributes to the behavior of a chemical substance by bonding with others to create molecules. When enough molecules come together, and are surrounded by light and information, they can form a living cell (*Universidad Finis Terrae* n.d.).

Every cell possesses an invisible energy field. The more organized this field is, the healthier the cell will be. Groups of similar cells form tissues: connective, epithelial, muscular, and nervous. Connective tissue supports and binds other tissues such as bone, blood, and lymph. These tissues work in coordination, thanks in part to the magnetic fields they emit.

Cells of the same tissue unite to form organs. Each organ holds an energetic field that carries the memory of that organ's function. Together, these organs form systems: digestive, reproductive, immune, cardiovascular, nervous, and musculoskeletal. Each of these systems draws from its own magnetic field to operate harmoniously and maintain balance.

When all systems work together, they create a unified body, with its own magnetic field. By interacting with the body's internal and external energetic resources, we can change the instructions stored within that field, helping the body respond to new conditions. We are energy. Tending to our magnetic field daily is vital, as it helps us counteract the constant energetic disturbances we encounter in modern life.

When cells lack adequate energy, their internal communication begins to break down. Without sufficient information or energy, the cell can no longer function and eventually dies.

Viewed at the atomic level, the human body resembles the universe, mostly composed of energetically charged empty space. Energy surrounds us constantly, and we can align with it to nurture our health.

The Law of Attraction tells us that like attracts like. We are energetic magnets, capable of charging and attracting everything around us, just as we attune ourselves to the things we desire. Our magnetic energy is self-governed; no one else can think or feel for us. It is through our thoughts and emotions that we create our frequency.

"The Universal Mind is not only intelligence, but substance, and that substance is the force of attraction that groups electrons by the law of attraction to form atoms: the atoms then group thanks to that same law to form molecules: the molecules adopt objective forms and we find the law is the creative force behind all manifestation, not only of atoms, but of worlds, of the universe, of all things that the imagination can conceive." —Charles Haanel (Haanel, 2017)

We are all energy fields. Quantum mechanics confirms this, as does quantum cosmology. The way we use this energy, whether positively or negatively, affects both our health and our environment. We are the creators of our own lives and, by extension, contributors to the unfolding of the universe. There is no limit to what human potential can achieve through focused energy, magnetic alignment, and conscious manifestation.

We are all connected, even if we cannot see it. Just like Wi-Fi, invisible yet undeniably real, energy binds the universe together.

> We have the ability to focus on internal well-being, regardless of external circumstances. Because we are energy, chiropractic care plays a vital role in maintaining the body's functionality.

The law established by Dr. Ralph U. Sierra in 1952 to regulate chiropractic practice in Puerto Rico and create the Puerto Rico Board of Chiropractic Examiners defines chiropractic as:

"The science of the treatment of the human body through adjustments and manipulations aimed at correcting deviations and partial dislocations of the spinal column which exert pressure on the nerves, hindering the transmission of vital energy from the brain to the organs, tissues, and cells of the human body."

The body is energy. That energy flows throughout us, influencing every aspect of our health and function. Chiropractic therapy can help restore or enhance any area of energetic stagnation in our personal magnetic field.

Long before he delved into biomagnetism or developed magnetic therapy, Dr. Ralph Sierra understood the immense energetic potential of the human being. He knew that we are not only surrounded by energy, we *are* energy, just like everything else in existence.

The History

In the 17th century, Isaac Newton formulated the law of universal gravitation, establishing that all material objects in the universe exert a gravitational pull on one another (The Editors of Encyclopaedia Britannica, 2024). According to this principle, every particle with mass attracts every other particle with mass through a force proportional to their masses and inversely proportional to the square of the distance between them.

In 1820, Hans Christian Ørsted, a physics professor in Copenhagen, discovered a relationship between electricity and magnetism. He observed that an electric current passing through a wire generated a magnetic field around it, which disappeared when the current stopped (*July 1820: Oersted and Electromagnetism*, n.d.). The magnetic field around a current-carrying wire could attract iron or metallic objects.

Building on these findings, Michael Faraday later introduced the concept of a *force field* (Faraday, Michael; Royal Society [Great Britain], n.d.). One of his most well-known experiments used iron filings to show the invisible lines of force surrounding a magnet. These filings arranged themselves along the magnetic field lines, illustrating how the field shapes the behavior and positioning of matter.

> This visualization revealed that magnetic fields do not require physical contact to exert influence; rather, they create a region around themselves—a field—within which their effects can be felt.

In 1831, Faraday made a groundbreaking discovery: magnetism could generate electricity. He demonstrated that moving a magnet near a coil of conductive wire induced an electric current in the wire, even without a battery. This led to the principle of electromagnetic induction. Eventually, scientists confirmed that electric and magnetic fields are part of a unified system, and James Clerk Maxwell expanded upon this understanding by concluding that light itself is a transverse vibration within this shared medium. He called it the electromagnetic field, a force field capable of generating both electrical and magnetic phenomena through its own oscillations.

For more than fifty years now, physics has expanded its view beyond matter and particles alone, recognizing the vital role of energetic fields, including the human energetic field, in the interaction of systems. Despite this evolution, Western medicine remains largely grounded in a mechanistic model. In biology, we continue to focus primarily on matter, often neglecting the energetic and wave-based dimensions that are essential to a more complete understanding of life and health.

The Science That Explains it

Our planet is surrounded by a terrestrial magnetic field. This field originates from Earth's geophysical structure, specifically its partially liquid core made of nickel and iron. As this molten core rotates, it generates the planet's magnetic field, which measures approximately 0.5 gauss. As human beings, we are constantly exposed to this natural magnetic influence. Beyond Earth, both the Sun and the Moon also have their own electromagnetic fields (EMFs), which affect not only our planet but the entire solar system.

Magnetism begins at the atomic level. As atomic electrons spin, they generate individual magnetic fields, causing each atom to behave like a tiny magnet. The difference between an unmagnetized and a magnetized iron bar lies in the alignment of these atomic magnets: in a magnet, they are arranged in an orderly fashion. All atoms have magnetic force and a field of influence. When they bond into molecules, they create a force field, an electromagnetic interaction that helps hold matter together.

Dr. Ralph U. Sierra explored these interactions by working directly with the electromagnetic field of cells through electromagnetic therapy. He discovered that combining chiropractic adjustments with electromagnetic energy, delivered via pulsed fields, could stimulate and vibrate every cell in the body. This allowed electromagnetic energy to reach all tissues, organs, and systems, saturating the entire body with what he called quantum energy: a force that provides light, information, and order. In Sierra's view, the human being is a microscopic version of the universe.

> It is important to recognize that the human body is more than just a complex arrangement of organs and chemical reactions. There is a vital force that animates us, one that Hippocrates referred to as *Vis Matura Medicatrix*—an inner power responsible for maintaining health and vitality.

There are several sources of magnetic fields in biological systems:

1. The magnetic poles associated with the atoms and molecules that make up our cells.

2. The magnetic fields generated by electric currents in active tissues, or as a result of activities like heartbeat, brain function, muscle contractions, etc.

While these magnetic fields are weak, they can be detected using tests such as electrocardiograms (EKG), electroencephalograms (EEG), and electromyograms (EMG).

In 1911, Dutch physicist Heike Kamerlingh Onnes discovered that mercury, when cooled to -269°C, no longer resisted the passage of electrical current. This was the birth of superconductors, materials that conduct electricity without resistance under specific conditions. Just two years later, Onnes was awarded the Nobel Prize in Physics (The Nobel Prize in Physics 1913, n.d.).

Superconductors also exhibit a fascinating phenomenon: they repel magnetic fields, allowing them to levitate above a magnetic surface, as though supported by an invisible force.

The scientific field of biomagnetism emerged in the 1970s. It focuses on the detection and measurement of the magnetic fields generated by living beings, particularly humans. This was made possible by the development of superconducting instruments sensitive enough to detect these subtle signals, including magnetic resonance imaging (MRI) and the SQUID magnetometer.

The *SQUID* magnetometer, short for *Superconducting Quantum Interference Device,* can detect extremely weak magnetic fields produced by the heart, brain, and other bodily systems. Introduced in France in 1987, SQUID-based biomagnetometers have since been widely used in medical research and diagnostics. Their applications are broad and promising, including detecting abnormal brain activity in patients with epilepsy or dementia, mapping sensory functions in the brain, identifying cardiac arrhythmias without invasive procedures, and detecting magnetic contaminants in the lungs, among others.

From these innovations arose specific applications such as neuromagnetism, cardiomagnetism, and pneumomagnetism. It was during this period that the scientific paradigm began to shift. The dominance of Newtonian physics and the prioritization of matter began to wane. The human body came to be understood primarily as energy and information. Slowly, conventional medicine began aligning with principles that natural medicine had embraced for centuries.

Just as magnetic field lines guide iron filings into visible patterns around a magnet, our bodies also follow an energetic blueprint, a holographic image that guides the arrangement and function of matter within us.

Understanding how and why this works empowers us to integrate it into our daily lives. When we truly understand our bodies not merely as mechanical structures, but as intelligent energetic systems, we transform them from passive vehicles into powerful allies for wellness.

It brings me joy that you are holding this book, because it means you are seeking to know more about yourself.

Chi, Chakras & Aura

When we look inward, we discover various sources of energy that flow outward from the body. These include the meridians, chakras, and the aura, three key components of the body's energetic system. In simple terms, chakras draw energy into the body, meridians distribute that energy throughout the body, and the aura is the body's surrounding energy field.

Meridians are energy pathways that span the body. In traditional Chinese medicine, they are recognized as acupuncture points, interconnected to form a sophisticated network of vessels and meridians. This energetic network not only moves energy through the body but also mirrors our internal condition, offering insight into the health of our organs, tissues, and systems.

The chakras are energetic centers located along the body's midline. The word *chakra* comes from Sanskrit and means *wheel*, as these centers are envisioned as spinning wheels that gather and circulate energy.

Every human being naturally has an invisible biomagnetic field that allows us to function. This field is known as the aura, and it is composed of physical, mental, emotional, and spiritual layers. It is similar to a rainbow and communicates through vibrations with the energies of the universe. It has two purposes: it connects us to our inner self through our neuroendocrine system, and it connects us to the universal mind. It also keeps our physical body healthy as long as the vibrational frequencies are normal.

> To maintain an optimal level of health, it's important that the integrity of the aura that surrounds our body is in good condition.

The aura is similar to Earth's magnetic field, which extends into space. Each cell in our body has polarity, and it can transmit signals that affect neighboring cells. If a cell is sick, its condition reflects in the aura and can disrupt the electromagnetic energy on its path through space.

It's important to keep in mind that there is a source of energy in every system, whether it is an atom, the solar system, a human being, or the universe. This energy has its own patterns and a sense of flow that moves through negative and positive poles. To maintain or achieve balance and health, energy must flow freely through the fields to and from its source. When this equilibrium is achieved, the vital energies can satisfy all healing needs. In addition, this balance leads to deep concentration, relaxation, radiant health, and a great peace of mind. Energy balance is key to true holistic human health.

The state of our physical and mental body affects this energetic field. For centuries, this force has been known as Chi or prana, and it is important that it flows to maintain good health. Imbalances and blockages in the energetic flow can be caused by physical factors such as poor diet, consumption of chemical substances, or trauma, as well as by emotional or mental factors like bad news, the loss of loved ones, suffering, or negative thoughts.

Our energy fields can both positively or negatively influence our biological health. The Earth's magnetic field is essential for life and for maintaining optimal health.

Electromagnetic fields generated by electromagnetic radiation have been linked to cancer and other health problems (Electromagnetic Fields and Cancer, 2022). To counteract the negative effects of these fields, the static magnetic field can offer benefits to our health. Also, when we are inside buildings, we move away from Earth's magnetic field.

Supplementing our natural magnetism with magnets, such as those used in the alternative therapy I developed in my practice, helps us to restore the normal flow of Chi and balance our natural magnetism. This facilitates the body's self-healing and contributes to our well-being.

Cellular Voltage

ere I'll be speaking to you in slightly more technical terms. Be patient, because it will be worth it. Our organs are separated by membranes. In a similar way, inside our cells, separation is maintained through electrical charges. Our cells, and all living organisms, are direct current (DC) systems, powered by the movement of sodium and potassium ions that pass in and out of the cell membranes.

Normal, healthy cells have an electrical charge of approximately -70 millivolts (mV) across their membrane. This electrical gradient is critical for ion transport and for maintaining proper cellular metabolism.

Cellular metabolism is responsible for the exchange of oxygen and nutrients for cellular waste, as well as for the production of ATP energy. ATP (Adenosine Triphosphate) is the main energy carrier molecule in all living forms like bacteria, yeasts, molds, algae, plants, and animal cells.

The body's electrical system is the nervous system. In fact, modern medicine depends on electrical processes. Without electricity, we would not have diagnostic tools such as electrocardiograms (EKG), electroencephalograms (EEG), and electromyograms (EMG), which are used to measure electrical activity in the heart, brain, and muscles.

According to Otto Heinrich Warburg, Nobel Prize winner in 1931 (The Nobel Prize in Physiology or Medicine 1931, n.d.), the membrane of nerve and muscle cells functions similarly to a battery. At birth, a healthy cell has a charge between -70 mV and -90 mV. As we age, this charge gradually declines. By age seventy, it can drop to around -35 mV. It's like watching a battery lose its charge.

A mature cell typically holds a charge between -50 mV and -35 mV. The older or sicker the person, the more the cellular voltage drops, which causes cells to vibrate out of rhythm with each other. When a cell's voltage falls below 15 mV, it is considered diseased and no longer functions properly.

When the immune system is overwhelmed, it cannot defend the body against toxins. This problem is worsened by the intake of alcohol, nicotine, caffeine, and negative thoughts or heavy emotions. Together, these factors throw the body out of balance.

Any stressor such as oxygen or nutrient deficiency, toxicity, or inflammation can degrade the membrane potential from its optimal -70 mV. As the gradient weakens, sodium is less effectively pumped out of the cell, leading to edema (fluid retention) and swelling. Oxygen transport across the membrane is also compromised, and without sufficient oxygen, the cell cannot generate ATP. This weakens the sodium-potassium pump further, setting off a downward spiral of disordered cellular function and eventual cell degeneration.

When the body's electrical charge increases, sodium (Na^+) and calcium ions (Ca^{2+}) exit the cell and enter the bloodstream, while potassium (K^+) and magnesium (Mg^{2+}) from the blood diffuse back into the cells. This regulates electrolyte balance inside and outside the cell (potassium-sodium transport). The result is that calcium ions help maintain the blood's slightly alkaline pH of 7.33 to 7.4. Excess sodium is expelled from the cells, and ATP production improves as potassium levels rise (Pirahanchi et al., 2023).

The electrical charge of inflamed cells (those causing pain) is approximately +30 mV. When exposed to a pulsed magnetic field, these cells can return to a healthier charge of -90 mV, relieving pain in the process. Scarred or fibrotic cells with adhesions have a charge of around +15 mV, and due to the density of such tissue, stronger pulsed magnetic fields are needed to restore them to their optimal -70 mV. Degenerative or immunocompromised cells average -30 mV.

Today, we know that living cells are like batteries: the nucleus carries a positive charge, and the cytoplasm carries a negative charge. When cells are exposed to a range of electromagnetic oscillations, they can be recharged and rejuvenated. Each cell and cell component responds to different frequencies, so a spectrum of frequencies is needed.

Each cell that participates in healing the body vibrates at a specific frequency. Every atom in the universe, whether a grain of sand, a piece of steel, a plant, an animal, or an organ, resonates at a particular frequency. Our bodies, composed of countless atoms, are permeated by photons, electrons, and a general bioelectric energy.

> The way we care for our body—physically, emotionally, and mentally—determines how much negative frequency or toxicity we accumulate.

Cells affected by negative conditions vibrate lower than they should. When this inner disharmony lasts for months or years, it weakens the immune system, eventually leading to the manifestation of disease or imbalance.

Each cell has a tiny electric pump whose job is to deliver nutrients and expel toxins. Without sufficient energy, these pumps fail, leaving cells toxic and malnourished. When an infectious organism attacks, these cells have already lost their capacity to resist.

Any challenge to the cell, such as lack of oxygen or nutrients, affects the -70 mV potential, just like a car battery running out. Without oxygen, ATP cannot be produced, and the sodium-potassium transport fails. Sodium accumulates inside the cell, causing edema (accumulation of liquid in the body) and swelling. The millivolts (mV) drop, and the cell enters a downward cycle of degeneration. Like a line of dominoes, once balance is lost, previously healthy molecules begin to deteriorate.

As time passes and technology continues to advance, there is increasing concern that electromagnetic pollution will affect future generations.

However, when cells are recharged to levels between -70 mV and -110 mV, diseases such as cancer cannot progress.

What Are The Benefits?

The cells within all human beings need to exercise. We can all benefit from the type of total cellular body exercise that magnetic therapy provides. This therapy can improve damaged areas of the cell and address the energy deficiency that causes chronic pain. A decrease in pain can be experienced as soon as after the first session.

By restoring the gradient, the cell begins to pump out sodium, allowing potassium to enter. This reduces inflammation, restores oxygen flow, and improves pain.

All cells exposed to the frequencies emitted by the pulsed magnetic field can lightly stretch and relax—in other words, they exercise.

Water is essential for expelling many of these toxins from the body. A good habit everyone should adopt is to drink plenty of water before and after exposure to a pulsated electromagnetic field to ensure optimum cellular hydration.

I recommend drinking two to three liters of water a day while using the pulsated magnetic field.

Static Magnetism Applied to Magnetic Therapy

As we've discussed previously, the north pole of a magnet is the negative and alkaline pole. This side of the magnet is much more healing and healthy. It has the ability to reduce acidity, body aches (such as headaches, glaucoma, and even menstrual pains), inflammations, hardening of the arteries, and it's even beneficial as a treatment for arthritis.

The blood's chemistry changes when it's exposed to magnets. When the magnet is used appropriately and at the correct frequencies, both poles can offer positive benefits. However, the function of the south pole is to stimulate, which may provoke a propagation of the very problem being treated.

Due to this, the positive south pole is considered detrimental and is generally avoided. Even in cases where patients claim that energy from the positive south pole has helped, there are often many other interfering factors. For instance the magnet's strength or gauss rating might be extremely low or inaccurate, causing no real effect, which could then be misinterpreted as improvement.

We must also confirm that the magnet has balanced poles. If we apply what we believe is the positive south pole of a magnet that is actually more magnetized with the negative north pole, it would not truly represent positive south pole energy. And, of course, the placebo effect cannot be ruled out either.

The Effects of Magnetic Poles

(N-)

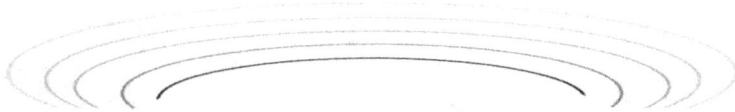

NORTH POLE **NEGATIVE**	SOUTH POLE **POSITIVE**
Relaxes	Stimulates
Reduces or alleviates pain	Increases pain
Produces more alkalinity	Acidifies
Reduces inflammation	Increases inflammation
Oxygenates cells	Decreases oxygen to cells
Attacks infections	Worsens infections
Promotes mental lucidity	Causes confusion
Reduces insomnia	Causes hyperactivity
Reduces fat accumulation	Increases fat accumulation
Regulates body functions	Stimulates body functions

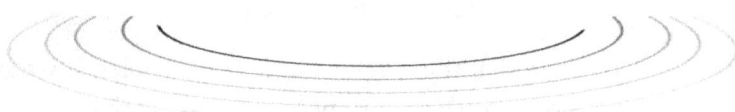

(S+)

Know Your Magnet

Intensity

The gauss is the unit of measurement used to express the strength of a magnetic field, much like the volt is used to measure voltage. Because magnets typically aren't sold with their gauss value labeled, and gaussmeters can be expensive, we need an alternative way to estimate the approximate strength. In general, the higher the gauss, the stronger the magnet.

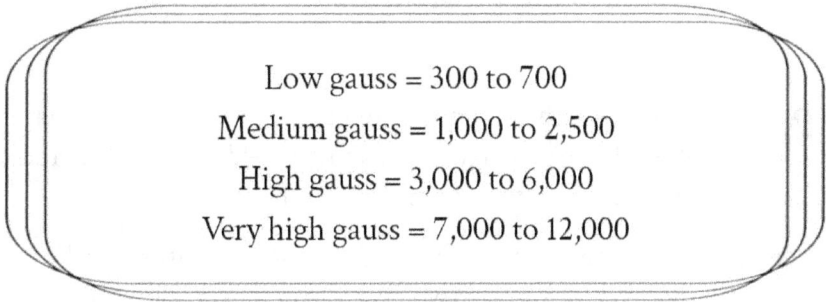

Low gauss = 300 to 700
Medium gauss = 1,000 to 2,500
High gauss = 3,000 to 6,000
Very high gauss = 7,000 to 12,000

Common units in nature

- 10.9 to 10.8 gauss – The human brain's magnetic field
- 0.31 to 0.58 gauss – Earth's surface natural magnetic field
- 25 gauss – Earth's core magnetic field
- 50 gauss – Typical fridge magnet
- 800 to 1,800 gauss – a small, disc-shaped ferrite magnet
- 2,500 gauss – one small neodymium-iron-boron magnet (NIB)
- 3,700 to 3,850 gauss – ferrite magnets, with ceramic grade 5 and 8 being the strongest.
- 11,000 gauss – samarium cobalt magnet (SmCo) (2:17 grade)
- 12,500 gauss – Alnico magnet (AlNiCo)
- 13,000 gauss – neodymium magnet (NdFeB) (N42 grade)
- 24,000 to 70,000 gauss – a medical magnetic resonance imaging machine

As a standard reference, I use 3,850 gauss permanent ceramic magnets, rated as N-1, N-2, N-3, in domino style with a 5-inch cylinder as the test unit, and 2,500 gauss magnetic points as our static magnets.

The list also includes wraps, bands, supports (braces) and accessories that contain ferrite or neodymium magnets ranging from 800 to 2,500 gauss, offering a practical alternative for daily use. Our magnets are always properly identified by pole. When using them, make sure to check the polarity beforehand. Remember to specifically use the negative north pole.

Depth

A magnet's strength can be affected by its size. While the gauss index itself doesn't change, the magnetic field can either increase or decrease depending on the dimensions of the magnet.

When used for treatment on the body, depth of penetration can be significantly enhanced by joining two ceramic magnets, allowing for a deeper therapeutic reach. A 3,800 gauss magnet can reach depths of up to 18 inches.

In many cases, even a pair of 0.25-inch thick magnets placed over a localized area can be more than enough for effective application.

General rule for choosing the magnet for magnetic therapy application

1 inch into the body = 200 gauss

2 inches into the body = 500 gauss

4 inches into the body = 1,500 gauss

6 inches into the body = 2,500 gauss

8 inches into the body = 3,500 gauss

For diseases or infections, the depth of the location site within the body should be 3 to 10 inches from the surface. This allows us to calculate the necessary magnetic negative energy of the north pole in gauss units and fortify the target area with a maximum of 2,500 to 4,000 gauss. Because energy is lost with distance, we must apply a greater amount of energy at the surface in order to reach the desired internal location. Additionally, it's important to keep in mind the amount of time the magnets are used—both the daily duration and the length of each application. The body needs time to register, process, and either soothe or stimulate the energy it receives through the blood's barrier and the entire system, especially in the area of the magnet placement.

Numbers

Magnets can't duplicate energy by being combined with other magnets. For example, a magnet with a gauss value of 500 will still have the same value when placed alongside an identical magnet (they do not combine to form 1,000 gauss). However, in this case, the magnetic field will expand.

A large number of magnets used together increases the depth and penetration of the magnetic field. When magnets are placed inside a pad or magnetic support, the more magnets it contains, the wider the magnetic field it will cover.

Space

The smaller the space between the magnet and the skin, the more effective the treatment will be. The beneficial effects of magnets come from the negative north pole, which is believed to increase the amount of oxygen available to the cells and create a more alkaline environment in the body. This contributes to faster healing in cases of cuts, broken bones, infections, and chronic illnesses like cancer.

Negative north pole energy may extend the lifespan of living systems by slowing down the aging process. It produces an effect of attraction and deceleration throughout the body. Application time should be carefully monitored.

Correct Management of the Positive South Pole

The positive south pole of a magnet should never be applied to a sore, swollen, infected, or diseased area, as this can worsen the condition.

This pole stimulates energy and increases vital activity. For example, since germs are a form of life, the energy from the positive south pole may actually promote their growth and development.

In more general terms, the energy from the positive south pole can strengthen muscles, extremities, joints, tendons, and ligaments. It also increases blood flow, promotes circulation and glandular activity, and stimulates the production of body fluids. This is the positive energy that supports and nourishes life.

Water that has been polarized with the positive south pole can be used to water houseplants, promoting strong and healthy growth.

Static Magnet Therapy

These are the magnets used in Dr. Sierra's magnetic bands, knee braces, pads, and N-1 and N-2 magnets. This type of therapy produces a static magnetic field that, in addition to relieving pain, may help the body restore its natural magnetism. When the body receives what it needs, it can achieve and maintain its internal balance, also known as homeostasis.

Compared to PEMF (Pulsed Electromagnetic Field) therapy, the success of therapy using static magnets alone depends on the strength of the magnets and the length of time they are applied. I use ferrite magnets, which are original permanent magnets. Time of use is important and varies depending on the case.

I've prepared a set of wellness magnets that can be used to perform magnetic therapy at home. The set includes one N-2 magnet, two N-1 magnets, two hand cylinders, a neck band, and an eye shield.

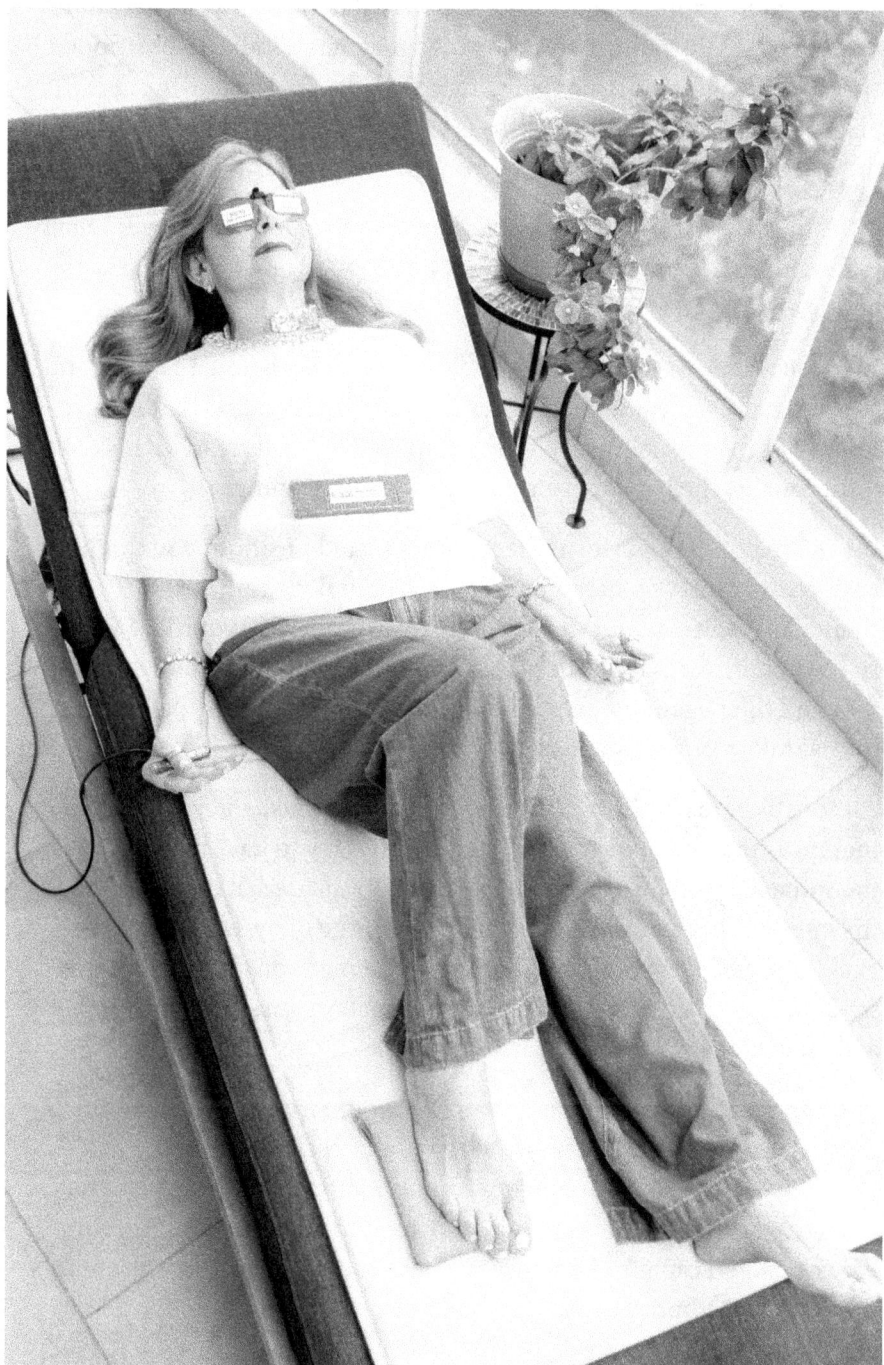

To use them while lying down, prepare a flat area on your bed and use a low, comfortable neck pillow. All magnets should be positioned with the negative north pole facing the body. Once everything is in place, lie down. Position each N-1 magnet under each shoulder and the N-2 magnet in the middle of your lower back, comfortably.

If the magnets feel too intense and you wish to place a layer over them, it should be as thin as possible so as not to interfere with the therapeutic effect.

Position the neckband and eye shield respectively below the neck and above the eyes. Take each cylinder in your hands and relax for a minimum of fifteen minutes, up to forty-five minutes. Try to do this daily. Additionally, the band can also be used while sleeping.

If you are going to perform therapy in a seated position, you can place both N-1 magnets on the floor and the N-2 under a thin cushion on the chair. This way, you can sit on top of the N-2 and rest your feet on each N-1. Another variation is to place the positive south pole under the left foot and the negative north pole under the right foot, while holding the cylinders in your hands.

Although these are the positions I recommend, the benefit of magnetic therapy is that it allows for variation. Always try to have a magnet near the spine. Depending on where the magnet is placed, it can affect multiple nerves that extend to different parts of the body. If placed on the neck, the treatment can reach the arms. Placing it on the thoracic area sends waves to the ribs, chest, or abdominal organs. Over the lumbar area, it can benefit the intestines and legs.

You can position the magnets wherever your situation requires them most. The N-1 magnets can be placed under each knee, on the ankles, or any area of the legs where you feel discomfort. They can also be applied to the abdomen, solar plexus, or used to treat gastric disorders. The neckband can also be worn as a headband. You may use the N-2 magnet on the upper back.

Be aware that if you suffer from any chronic pain condition and begin using static magnets or PEMF therapy, you may experience a temporary worsening of symptoms. This period typically lasts between 24 to 48 hours, due to the initial impact the magnets have on the affected area. It's similar to when you fracture your ankle and receive a cast. The first few days are always the most uncomfortable. It's not that the therapy isn't working. Sometimes, healing involves a bit of discomfort.

Magnetic Jewelry

In 1954, Dr. Linus Pauling received the Nobel Prize for discovering that hemoglobin has magnetic properties (The Nobel Peace Prize 1962, n.d.). Pauling found that iron and many electrolyte salts in our blood circulate biomagnetically. This discovery helps explain why the continuous proximity of a magnetic field can accelerate circulation and energy transfer throughout the body.

Magnetic jewelry is a convenient way to benefit from magnetic therapy on a daily and mobile basis. Ralph U. Sierra was a pioneer in promoting its use, and this was part of the reason we founded our *Health Magnetic Store & More*. We wanted to ensure that this type of therapeutic magnet would be accessible and reliably manufactured. The magnetic jewelry we offer is made with neodymium magnets.

Neodymium magnets are strong and durable, similar to biomagnets. These are high-intensity magnets not commonly available in non-specialized stores. With proper care, they can last more than fifty years. My family has been using magnetic jewelry for over five decades for treating patients, animals, and even plants. Magnetic jewelry is made using negative north pole energy.

The purpose of wearing magnetic jewelry, whether a necklace, bracelet, ring, or ankle bracelet, is to strengthen and keep the body's cells constantly charged. These items provide energy to the cells, which need it to function optimally. Magnetic jewelry also helps counteract the effects of harmful and negative electromagnetic radiation, such as that emitted by cell phones, wireless signals, electrical appliances, and steel structures.

For example, if your wrist, hand, or arm hurts, you may be experiencing muscular spasms in those areas. Depending on the duration and severity of the pain, whether it radiates or causes tingling, you may benefit from wearing a bracelet on each wrist. The magnetic field can help increase circulation in your wrists, hands, and fingers as it moves through the blood and into the rest of the body. Magnetic jewelry can be worn twenty-four hours a day, seven days a week, for best results.

> Remember that negative ions support the reduction of inflammation and pain, help combat stress, and increase both energy and oxygen flow to the brain, which improves alertness.

Stainless steel and titanium bracelets typically have at least eight links, each containing a 3,000 gauss magnet. Stainless steel rings contain three magnets of 2,000 gauss each. Jewelry is available in a variety of styles for both polarities.

This is a non-invasive therapy. There are no injections, and no pills to take. It acts as a sedative for the nerves, helping to relieve pain and promote muscular relaxation.

Fortunately, science now recognizes that animal and plant cells share many similarities with electric batteries. Your body has always contained electricity, and PEMF therapy and magnetic therapy are simply the reconciliation of that fact. We now have a therapeutic method that allows us to cultivate and stimulate the energy that is already within us. As Sierra often said, "we are energy."

Memory Band

Sierra's memory band helps normalize mental abilities. This can result in improved information retention, a reduction in depression, and an amplification of psychic abilities. The band is made with a one-inch flexible magnetic strip of high energy, designed to stimulate the north (front of the head) and south (back of the head) poles.

Attaching the negative north pole of a magnet to the center of the forehead for ten minutes a day increases the brain's perception and sensitivity. This amplifies psychic abilities and also helps relieve stress and the pressure caused by daily demands, allowing the brain to function more effectively.

Because the frontal lobe regulates memory, emotions, behavior, and decision-making functions, using the band daily can help minimize depression, improve emotional regulation, and support the treatment of behavioral disorders. The back of the band directs energy through the occipital lobe. The magnets can also be interchanged if considered necessary and beneficial.

These positive effects are tangible for a limited time. To maintain the stimulation that makes these effects possible, consistent application of the magnet to the forehead is required. Over time, the mind becomes so alert that it not only experiences stimulation, but may also enter a state of mystical awareness.

Thanks to Dr. Robert Becker (Becker & Marino, 1982) and physicist Charles Bachmans (CH. B., 1962), we know that the energy we emit and the emotional changes we experience are influenced by electromagnetic and chemical shifts in the brain and spinal cord nerves. These shifts are affected by geomagnetic fluctuations. Scientists explain that the electric field alternates from positive to negative and then naturally returns to its negative state during the healing process.

It is recommended not to exceed three thirty-minute sessions, with the north magnet on the forehead and the south on the back of the head. It's fine if you go over this time, but be mindful of how you feel. Experiment with each polarity and observe the effects.

I encourage you to learn more about how your brain and body can unlock their full potential while using magnetic bands. Expanding your knowledge will bring great benefits to your overall well-being.

If you can only apply the band once a day, here's a helpful trick for your nighttime routine: place the magnetic band or a small magnet on the area where the bridge of the nose meets the forehead. This spot corresponds to the third eye. Keep it in place for ten to fifteen minutes before bed.

Of course, this isn't the only way to use magnets on the body. Magnets can be applied to any area you wish, as long as you keep the rules of polarity and their effects in mind. Speaking from experience, the first time my father treated me with magnets, it was for an earache using a domino-shaped magnet. He then used an N-1 negative north pole magnet on my abdomen to relieve a terrible stomach ache.

We used to call the N-1 our "home doctor," and I still stand by that playful expression. There was a time I suffered from menstrual cramps and heavy periods. Since I was in school, I couldn't use the N-1 during the day, and I was too restless at night. So it took me a little longer to feel relief, but I did, and I never had that pain again.

Today, we have a net-like band with eight magnets that women can place between their underwear and lower abdomen to relieve menstrual pain at any time. That way, they don't have to wait as I once did.

I learned to sleep with the magnetic neckband as a teenager. Even now, if I feel tension building, the first thing I do is put it on. I wear it most of the time while I'm at home. My sons, daughter, and now my grandchildren are all accustomed to wearing the magnetic band regularly.

My father also participated in the research that led to the creation of a magnetic hairbrush. He attached a domino-shaped magnet with positive south pole energy to a regular brush to strengthen and stimulate the scalp and hair follicles. Brushing your hair at night helps discharge the positive ions accumulated from stress and recharges the body using the magnetic brush.

I personally credit the health of my hair to those brushes I grew up with and still use. They're so effective that we continue to offer them to patients and clients. They're manufactured the same way Sierra originally made them, nothing has changed.

Even after years of hair treatments and dyeing, my hair remains perfectly healthy and shiny. Even my husband's hair is in excellent condition. The positive south pole strengthens the scalp, while the negative north pole can be applied to any part of the body that needs relaxation or calming. My father also recommended magnetic inserts for the feet.

Polarized Water

The water we drink can be magnetized. After one of his trips to the Albert Roy Davis Laboratory in Green Cove Springs, my father brought back an additional N-2 magnet, which he placed underneath the water jug in our refrigerator. He also brought back Davis's knowledge about magnetizing water for plants and decided to implement it at home as well.

At first it was just a magnet placed under the refrigerator, with the north pole (negative) facing up toward the jug. Later, he found a five-inch ceramic cylinder that perfectly held the jug on top. So, by the time I was eight years old, I was drinking water that had been polarized with negative ions. Eventually, he also included the magnetic stir stick so we could magnetize our drinks even when we weren't at home.

Water that has been exposed to the negative north pole should always be used for human or animal consumption. Sierra discovered that water magnetized with the north negative pole has greater surface tension. This makes the water harder and heavier due to increased hydrogen ion activity and reduced levels of dissolved oxygen and nitrogen.

Drinking water magnetized with the negative north pole can have therapeutic effects. Magnetized water has an alkalizing and oxidizing effect, which can influence chemical hypersensitivity. Most of the toxins in the body are acidic, and this acidity can be reduced thanks to the alkalizing properties of magnetized water.

Water magnetized with the south pole, on the other hand, has lower surface tension. It becomes softer water, so soft that it's even softer than untreated water. This water is especially useful for plants, as it speeds up their growth and allows proteins to be absorbed more easily through the roots than with regular water. This type of water increases the nutritional value of edible plants and improves their taste. It also enhances the mineral content in soil.

Any water container can be magnetically treated. All you need to do is place the container on top of a magnetic cylinder for any amount of time. Drinking this water throughout the day supports the body's daily functions.

If you want to magnetize the water supply of an entire house, you can do it by attaching one or two north pole (negative) magnets to the pipe that carries the water into the home. About two inches above that, attach one or two south pole (positive) magnets. The number of magnets will depend on the size of the pipe.

Another method for polarizing water with both polarities is using the magnetic pencil. Just place the magnetic pencil in a glass of water for three to ten minutes. If you want to magnetize your water with only one polarity, either north or south, fill a 32 oz to 64 oz glass container and place it on top of a flat ceramic magnet. Let it sit for twelve to twenty-four hours. If possible, leave the container on top of the magnet and keep refilling it as you drink. A good habit is to fill it up before bed, so the water polarizes overnight.

If you want to magnetize bottled water, place a flexible magnet on a cup holder and set the bottle on top. Depending on the bottle's size, the water will be magnetized in ten to fifteen minutes. Once magnetized, polarized water retains its properties for up to three days.

I learned how to do this from my father, who confirmed Albert Roy Davis' experiments with water and plants. Water treated with magnets showed noticeable differences compared to untreated water in terms of minerals, solids, pH, and other elements. However, although the hydrogen amounts were the same, the hydrogen ions in the magnetized water were altered and demonstrated a much higher level of activity. These results were consistent in repeated tests.

Water treated with either the north or south magnetic field tends to reduce nitrogen levels. This makes it safer for both human consumption and aquarium fish.

Magnetic Field Deficiency

Researchers such as Dr. Kyoichi Nakagawa believe that magnetic field deficiency syndrome occurs due to a decrease in the Earth's magnetic field. This syndrome is characterized by symptoms such as fatigue, insomnia, frequent headaches, dizziness, and generalized aches and pains (Nakagawa, 1976).

Our modern lifestyle also contributes to this condition. Many of us spend most of our time inside steel buildings and metal vehicles, limiting our exposure to the Earth's natural magnetic field. This disruption in energy flow can alter cellular metabolism. And if our cells aren't functioning well, the body won't be either, whether as a whole or in its individual parts.

For this reason, we recommend applying an external magnetic field to the human body to compensate for magnetic deficiency. In summary, there is a direct relationship between the decrease in the Earth's magnetic field and the improvement of abnormal conditions in the body through the application of external magnetic fields.

> This magnetic deficiency syndrome can be reversed or even avoided by ensuring the body receives adequate exposure to direct current (DC) magnetism. This can be achieved by providing the body with either a static or pulsating magnetic field through magnet therapy.

A simple way to do this is by wearing magnetic jewelry. Once the body's magnetic field returns to a balanced state, also known as homeostasis, the symptoms of magnetic deficiency tend to disappear, and health can be restored.

Pulsed Electromagnetic Field Therapy (PEMF)

ave you ever held two magnets in your hands and tried to push them together? You probably felt them repel each other, and no matter how hard you tried, you couldn't make them touch. If you've felt that, then you've experienced what magnetic fields feel like.

The Earth has its own magnetic field, which exists due to changes in the planet's core. Compasses are able to identify the direction of the north (negative) and south (positive) poles thanks to this electromagnetic field, produced by moving electric charges. This field affects any object within its range. It is a natural activity of the universe.

Pulsed Electromagnetic Field therapy, better known as PEMF, is used to improve circulation and cellular metabolism. In Puerto Rico, this therapy is known primarily thanks to Dr. Ralph U. Sierra. My family and I continue to share his legacy in our chiropractic clinics.

PEMF therapy penetrates at the cellular level, where it causes the desired stimulation. This magnetic field passes through the body as if the magnetic frequencies were gusts of wind. These low frequencies travel through the skin to promote cellular metabolism, reduce inflammation, improve circulation, and balance the immune system. In addition, they relax and repair muscles, bones, tendons, and stimulate the organs.

The main goal of PEMF therapy is to accelerate the healing process from the inside out. These are just a few of the benefits that can be observed after a few PEMF treatments. A study conducted by NASA

(Goodwin, 2006) demonstrated that this therapy significantly stimulates tissue growth and repair, improves cellular function, and has modulating effects on certain neurodegenerative diseases.

Dr. Ralph U. Sierra manufactured copper coils to administer electromagnetic therapy in the 1970s. As a doctor, a chiropractor, and throughout my life, I have received and used this therapy, which is still offered at Jarrot Sierra Chiropractic Clinic. Thanks to the passage of time and advances in technology, new PEMF therapy equipment has been developed, so much so that if you don't want to go elsewhere to receive therapy, you can have a PEMF machine in your home.

Is PEMF therapy better than static magnets? The question is not whether one treatment is better than the other, but rather how the treatments compare. PEMF is another form of therapy that involves receiving a magnetic field, but in this one, the electricity produces cellular vibration, a greater and more dynamic effect. A static magnet has a fixed magnetic field, it doesn't change. However, PEMF generates a magnetic field by conducting electricity through a set of copper coils inside the applicator (usually a mat). Therefore, PEMF does not require static magnets. This process produces a much larger and more dynamic magnetic field. Since PEMF is an electromagnetically induced magnetic field, its effect is achieved by transferring charge to the body's cells.

A pulsed electromagnetic field can penetrate the entire body and create a cascade of positive effects. Because it is a dynamic field, the body does not become accustomed to the magnetic field, allowing long-term treatments to be truly effective. PEMF treatments can be shorter than static magnet treatments, and the magnetic field intensity can be significantly lower. Still, it produces similar effects within the body.

PEMFs are a wellness and fitness device. They are not targeted to a specific disease.

Benefits of PEMF Therapy

- Enhancement of self-repair mechanisms
- Improved tissue oxygenation
- Improved blood circulation and blood pressure
- Improved muscle function and physical performance
- Pain reduction and decreased inflammation
- Energizes cells so they can function properly
- Stimulates bone repair
- Decreases inflammation and swelling
- Strengthens the immune system
- Acts as a natural pain reliever while healing tissue
- Used to treat symptoms of arthritis and other chronic pain conditions
- Enhances wound healing
- Increases energy
- Improves nutrient absorption
- Balances acupuncture meridians

Intensity

Intensity is the strength, amplitude, or quantity of the signal delivered by the machine. The therapy will be effective regardless of whether the electromagnetic energy is low, medium, or high. The intensity of a magnetic field is commonly measured in gauss or microtesla (100 microtesla = 1 gauss). The "charge" that is therapeutically induced in the stimulated tissues depends on the intensity of the magnetic field.

For example, to treat areas of the body where the skin is thick, higher intensity electromagnetic energy would be needed. The same principle can be applied in cases involving casts, orthopedic braces, and fractures. There is no exact way to determine which intensity would be beneficial for each body area or treatment, so it is important to gather as much information as possible to properly experiment with intensities.

Frequency

> *"If you want to find the secrets of the universe, think in terms of energy, frequency and vibration."*
>
> —*Nikola Tesla*

Frequency refers to the number of pulses the signal emits per second, and it is measured in Hertz. The unit was named in honor of German physicist Heinrich Rudolf Hertz, the first person to definitively prove the existence of electromagnetic waves, the same waves predicted by an equation created by Scottish physicist James Clerk Maxwell.

Every type of cell can produce a unique response to a given frequency. Different frequencies can have different effects on the body. Typically, PEMF (Pulsed Electromagnetic Field) therapy uses low frequencies and long waves ranging from 1 to 100 Hz, and sometimes up to 10,000 Hz.

In this context, we refer to the frequency of both energy ($E = hv$) and information. The field of energy medicine is increasingly focused on frequency, moving away from intensity as the main consideration. Although frequency is a bit more complex, it is essential for understanding both energy medicine and PEMF therapy.

Imagine frequency as a wave, pulse, or cycle that passes through a fixed location within a given time. If ten waves pass through a single point in one second, the frequency is ten cycles per second, or 10 Hz.

Frequencies are typically managed through pre-programmed settings that come with the machine, which is why it's important to determine what settings your body may need before purchasing a device.

For example, low-frequency PEMF emits a magnetic field of medium to high intensity. This type of frequency is excellent for treating solid tissues such as bones. In contrast, high-frequency PEMF produces small, rapid pulses at low intensity, which are ideal for treating soft tissues such as muscles and tendons.

Applicators

The thicker the patient's skin, the more the intensity of the magnetic field is reduced. Ideally, the patient's skin should have direct contact with the source that emits the magnetic field, which in this case is the applicator.

Some PEMF units include full-body pillows that allow the user to recline or sit on them. These are designed to ensure that the entire body comes into contact with the PEMF coils. My advice is to be in contact with six to eight of these coils. They can be used for ten to thirty minutes, once or up to three times per day.

Polarity

Some machines are designed to change the direction of the magnetic pulse. This is known as a polarity change or magnetic inversion. It involves the reversal of the magnetic poles and the flow of the magnetic field, so that the positions of the negative north pole and the positive south pole are exchanged.

Different Types of Waves

1. **Sinusoidal wave**: This type of wave mimics the natural waves produced by the body.

2. **Square wave**: Beneficial for stimulating and regenerating cells. The shorter, sharper wave delivered through a mat or pillow

can penetrate the cells more easily, improve blood flow, and fine-tune the body's natural signals. This promotes quicker healing and tissue restoration.

3. **Sawtooth waveform:** A non-sinusoidal wave operating at low frequencies between 0.5 and 15 Hz. This frequency range falls entirely within the so-called "biological window." Unlike simple sinusoidal waves or static magnets, the sawtooth signal changes constantly, which continuously induces electromagnetism into body tissues. This helps maximize ion distribution and prevents fatigue in the cell membranes.

When using the system for the first time, it's best to start with ten-minute sessions. Intensity and time can be gradually increased as the patient adapts to the treatment. If there isn't a specific condition to treat, therapy can begin at the system's maximum time and intensity. Little (*petite*) or thin individuals, as well as children and animals, may be more sensitive to the treatment.

Each setting offers its own benefits. There are no wrong choices, since the system is designed to work at low intensity. In most cases, using the maximum intensity is recommended to provide the greatest benefit to the body.

For acute conditions, treatment time can be extended. There is no strict limit to how long the system can be used. If there are any concerns about sensitivity, it is advisable to start at 3 Hz with low intensity.

Preset Intensity, Frequency and Treatment Times

Many devices allow you to customize programs for specific treatments. Some only let you adjust the level of intensity and the duration of the session. It's essential to ensure you are using the program correctly.

For example, in my case, my personal frequency is 10 Hz for thirty minutes, and the program I use afterward fluctuates between 7.8 and 31 Hz. I receive both sinusoidal and square waves. I use an instrument the size of a pillow with a personalized program for when I travel, and it fits perfectly in a suitcase. Since it only covers the midsection of the body, I move it between my upper back, lower back, and legs. I always combine PEMF therapy with static magnets—N-1, N-2, N-3—hand cylinders, and I cover my eyes with magnetic shields for added support.

Some PEMF units also include preset programs with specific frequencies linked to different organ systems, chakras, and meridians. There are devices with personalized programs that allow you to choose any frequency from 0.1 Hz up to 99.9 Hz. Some include Theta frequencies (7 to 10 Hz) and Alpha frequencies (8 to 13 Hz). If you are sensitive, your initial treatments should use lower frequencies and shorter durations. I suggest starting with 4 Hz and gradually increasing to 7.8 Hz, which is the Earth's natural frequency (Schumann, 1952).

All of this can seem very technical, which is why I strongly recommend that you make these decisions with the guidance of a chiropractor or a healthcare professional who understands this science. That person will be best equipped to evaluate your specific needs and help you choose the equipment and programs that are right for you.

Magnet and PEMF therapy for autoimmune conditions is usually a lifelong practice. Magnetic therapy helps reduce inflammation and the intensity of the immune response, while also supporting tissue repair without side effects. My experience has shown that both static and pulsed magnetic therapy can lessen the severity and duration of flareups associated with autoimmune episodes. It also significantly reduces dysfunction and long-term damage to the organs.

The body is, in fact, a magnet, and by applying external magnetic fields, we can improve blood flow and treat inflammation.

Should You Buy a PEMF Machine?

Before purchasing a PEMF machine, take a moment to assess how much you need it. Consider whether you intend to use the device for personal use or for the entire family, as this will influence which type of machine and program options are most suitable. Your lifestyle, whether sedentary or active, can also help determine which machine is the most convenient for your needs. In cases of chronic or debilitating conditions, you may require additional types of stimulation or complementary therapies alongside electromagnetic treatment.

PEMF machines can be adapted to meet different physiological needs through various intensities and frequencies. Many models allow you to select from preset programs or modify the settings to personalize your therapy.

Always keep in mind that the ideal energy for the body is that which comes directly from the Earth: a dynamic energy with a frequency range between 0 and 30 Hz. The most suitable PEMF machine for you will be the one that aligns with the frequency your body responds to best and the waveform that delivers that energy effectively to your cells.

In 1995, Sisken and Walker found that a frequency of 2 Hz stimulates nerve regeneration. They also observed that 7 Hz promotes bone growth, 10 Hz supports ligament healing, and 15, 20, and 72 Hz can help reduce skin necrosis and stimulate the formation of capillaries. Since all tissues and organs are composed of cells, the human body resonates with and responds best to frequencies in the 0 to 30 Hz range (Sisken & Walker, 1995).

Devices with 15 gauss are suitable for short-term use, but not recommended as the foundation for long-term wellness. It's important to have a clear understanding of how often and for what purposes you plan to use your PEMF machine.

What to Expect During a Session

During a typical electromagnetic session, most people feel pulsations and a noticeable stimulation in the areas being treated. If you combine your PEMF therapy with a static magnet, you may feel vibrations when placing the magnet near the inner coil of the unit. This sensation is usually pleasant.

Of course, individual experiences may vary depending on several factors, including the specific equipment being used, the frequency applied, and the programming of the session.

How Does the Magnetic Field Affect the Body?

Magnetic fields can influence the behavior of everything around them. Each heartbeat generates electromagnetic waves that travel through the bloodstream, stimulating tissues at the cellular level.

> When an electromagnetic field moves through the entire body, it interacts with all seventy trillion of our cells. This stimulation encourages each cell to perform its specific function while helping to restore balance and minimize pain.

Magnetic fields positively affect the molecules and tissues of the body. Let's look at some of these effects:

1. **Energizing**: As part of their general role, cells generate energy, eliminate waste, repair, and regenerate. Depending on their type and location, they may also carry out additional functions. Electromagnetic fields directly stimulate the mitochondria, the energy centers of our cells, boosting their natural production of ATP (adenosine triphosphate). This increases the body's natural energy levels, allowing it to better resist illness and dysfunction.

2. **Balancing**: Magnetic fields elevate ion and electrolyte movement within tissues and bodily fluids, helping the body to re-balance and, when needed, to self-heal.

3. **Stimulating**: Even brief exposure to low-frequency pulsed electromagnetic fields can stimulate cellular metabolism, improve oxygen absorption, and speed up chemical detoxification. These fields can penetrate the body and naturally support its biological rhythms, enabling the body to recover and activate its self-healing abilities.

4. **Strengthening**: One long-term benefit of PEMF therapy is cellular protection. Electromagnetic fields help repair cells, improve circulation, and supply them with energy. They also increase the production of stress proteins, which help prevent

cell degradation and enhance the body's ability to recover. Magnetic fields contribute to the balance of cells, tissues, and bodily functions at a fundamental level and can help resolve health issues before the body fully assimilates them.

5. **Improves circulation**: PEMF therapy supports better blood flow throughout the vascular system, especially in the micro-capillaries—the smallest blood vessels in the body. Improved circulation enhances oxygenation in tissues and helps eliminate metabolic waste via healthy blood cells. Energized blood cells are then transported to all areas of the body, promoting faster recovery and a stronger immune response.

Recommendations

For general well-being, the use of static magnets and PEMF therapy is recommended at least twice a day for a minimum of fifteen minutes. This routine helps recharge your cells and support your body's natural balance.

Before beginning your therapy session, drink at least an eight-ounce glass of pure water. It's also advised to avoid smoking, consuming caffeine, or drinking alcohol immediately before or after your session. After the therapy, drink plenty of water, ideally eight to ten glasses of eight ounces each, or about two liters per day, to support hydration and assist with the detoxification process.

To maintain the positive effects of magnetic therapy, it's recommended to follow a clean diet free from chemicals, pesticides, and refined sugars. Eating plenty of green vegetables is encouraged.

PEMF machines can stimulate the body's antioxidant systems and may initiate a detox process. For that reason, it's helpful to stay well hydrated and support your body with supplements, multivitamins, and Omega oils, ideally using formulas designed for your specific condition.

Can I Learn to Lead a Magnetic Life?

"We now stand on the verge of a great new age in magnetic science and its applications, a tool that has been provided by Mother Nature itself."

— Dr. Ralph U. Sierra, 1978

"Discover magnetism [by] reaching out to nature's energy."

— Dr. Irma I. Sierra, 2004

Magnets to Live a Good Life

The use of magnets goes far beyond the everyday uses we've become accustomed to, like sticking them on the fridge or incorporating them into electronic accessories. Magnets can also be used to heal.

If you experience a migraine and hold the negative north pole of a magnet to the front of your head, the pain may ease and the migraine can improve. The same effect has been observed in cases of broken bones and chronic pain conditions like acute rheumatic pain. For over fifty years, I've proudly witnessed how magnets and their magnetic fields, especially the energy of the negative north pole and negative ions, positively affect all living things.

People who use magnetic therapy can attest to its powerful healing properties, whether for arthritis, migraines, injuries, or even cancer.

In an interview with Alicia Gutiérrez Moreno, my father, Dr. Ralph U. Sierra, shared the following:

"When we inhale air through our nose, we are charging our batteries. We're not just breathing in oxygen, we're absorbing the negative or positive charges in the environment. It's no coincidence that in yoga, practitioners are taught to draw energy to their point of concentration through deep breathing. This is entirely real. And if the power of magnetism was once obscured by academic prejudices, today we know that this magnetic energy represents life itself. It encompasses and governs everything, or at the very least, our form of terrestrial life. To talk about the effects of magnetism is to enter into the smallest and subtlest aspects of cellular life, human behavior, and life on this planet."

The more we tap into the magnetic field through magnets with the correct polarity and strength, the more we activate and harmonize biomagnetic energy. In doing so, we help the body—its cells, tissues, organs, and systems, all composed of atoms, molecules, and chemical interactions—restore and renew themselves.

Health Renewal

Recovering your health is not impossible, but it's not easy either. It's a long and challenging journey that requires deep understanding before you even begin. Anyone seeking to improve their health must first understand the root causes of their symptoms. Knowing what triggers your symptoms and what you are experiencing puts you in a better position to take control of your recovery in a meaningful and sustainable way.

Understanding why you feel the way you do gives you the motivation to seriously commit to a wellness program. Without that awareness, it's easy to lose interest or neglect your well-being. It's important to recognize that not all ailments come from medical conditions. Many are caused by lifestyle choices, or a combination of both. In any case, the message remains the same: recovering your health requires commitment.

After years of poor health, those who adopt positive changes to increase their vitality must go through a transition period. Just as chronic illness does not develop overnight, optimal health can't be achieved instantly. Even though society tends to favor quick fixes through medications or treatments, real and lasting relief comes from making lifestyle changes: eating well, applying electromagnetic therapy, and practicing other supportive habits. But this relief is directly tied to the consistency of those habits.

> It's essential not to abandon a health program just because you feel better after a few days, or because the improvement is slow. Health is built on consistent efforts that strengthen the body's vitality and its capacity for cellular regeneration.

In the beginning, improving your health may feel uncomfortable, even painful. But pushing through that discomfort is crucial if you want to experience long-term results.

There are two real options: keep looking for quick fixes that only treat symptoms and may cause side effects, or address the problem at its root.

This means changing your behavior and mindset, and committing to practices that strengthen your body so you can reach levels of wellness you may have never experienced before.

Many people get injured during exercise, household tasks, or physically demanding work. Sometimes these injuries are worsened by destructive habits such as poor diet, lack of sleep, alcohol or drug use, or emotional and psychological stress.

Whether intentional or not, these behaviors contribute to the buildup of waste inside and around the tissues of the body. Add to that the environmental factors we can't always control: pollution, electromagnetic radiation from microwaves, WiFi, antennas, electronic devices, pesticides, heavy metals, and more. It all accumulates, and the body holds on to it. That's the challenge.

To manage both the things we can and cannot control, the body must be maintained in a strong and balanced state. That's why conscious, ongoing maintenance is key to facing life's challenges with resilience and well-being, even during difficult times.

I recommend making consistent changes across various areas of your life, but it's also important to eventually reach a balance among them. For example, someone may eat well and manage stress effectively, but if they're still experiencing chronic inflammation, it can lead to nerve, joint, muscle, and organ issues, resulting in more serious conditions like diabetes, heart disease, Alzheimer's, or emotional disorders. Inflammation is often called "the silent killer." It can also lead to fatigue, skin problems, digestive issues, hormonal imbalances, and more.

It's normal to feel resistant or afraid of change. But what's not normal is knowing that change is necessary and doing nothing about it. The key is simply to try.

That's why I believe it's helpful to know the benefits of change, but even more important is to understand the challenge. You will likely encounter obstacles along the way, but where there is a will, there is always a way. It's like remodeling an old building. You have to tear down the outdated structure before rebuilding something stronger and more modern. The end result is worth it, even if the process feels messy and chaotic.

The most beautiful part of the path to wellness is that the more you maintain your practice, the fewer symptoms you'll feel. With time, you will feel better and may even experience the disappearance of some symptoms. Your body will improve.

But just as it takes time to develop illness, it will also take time to heal. The body needs space to rest, recharge, and eliminate the buildup of impurities that have accumulated over the years. Eventually, the discomfort will fade and be replaced by extended periods of wellness and inner peace.

At some point, you will reach a state of sustained well-being. You'll apply what you've learned, and you'll understand that living in harmony with the natural laws of health is the key. Falling back into bad habits will only lead you back to suffering the consequences of illness.

Here are some tips I consider essential for achieving full health and wellness. You may already practice some of them, but all are equally important and should be integrated consistently. These points are non-negotiable in my life:

- Drink pure, magnetically polarized water. Eliminate carbonated soft drinks and concentrated juices.

- Manage your stress, and in the process, change the way you visualize your world. Be happy, stay optimistic. Practice introspection. Pay attention to what you say and reflect on it. Don't believe every negative thought you have about yourself.

- Sleep seven to nine hours. Try to be in bed by 10:00 p.m. or earlier. This helps the body heal and makes the most of the critical window between bedtime and 2:00 a.m., when cortisol, melatonin, and insulin levels naturally recalibrate.

- Preserve your mental balance through patience and regular self-reflection.

- Incorporate meditation into your daily life. From the moment you wake until you fall asleep, envision a future that excites you. Don't dwell in the past, and don't let yesterday repeat itself today or tomorrow.

- Eat real, organic food. Avoid preservatives and chemicals. Try fasting occasionally (with guidance from a health professional), switch to a liquid diet temporarily, or make other informed nutritional adjustments.

- Choose herbal, organic supplements. Make sure they're free from GMOs and gluten.

- Use magnetic therapy regularly. Combine static magnets with PEMF therapy when possible. Close your eyes, breathe deeply, and relax—let the magnets support your healing.

- Breathe slowly and with intention.

- Sunbathe and spend time outdoors. As living beings, we need the radiation the sun provides. Moderate sun exposure strengthens the immune system and helps the body produce vitamin D. Always use sunscreen.

- Connect with nature. Start a garden. Spend time near plants. Walk barefoot on the grass or sand. Hug a tree.

- Step away from technology as much as possible.

- Move your body through Chi energy exercises such as Qi-gong, Tai Chi, yoga, or Reiki. Your body is meant to move, so move it! Explore color therapy, sound healing, crystals, and chakra balancing.

- Heal spiritual wounds. Be at peace with yourself and in your relationships.

- Live in the present moment. Practice presence.

- Visit your chiropractor regularly for spinal adjustments, and combine the treatment with cold laser therapy and massage if needed.

- Raise your hands to the universe and express gratitude. Be thankful for everything, good and bad. Everything happens for a reason.

- Love life. Find love in everything.

Your efforts to restore your health and live in alignment with nature's laws may feel like a lot at first—but over time, they reveal what true health really means: the ability to enjoy your life and make a positive impact on the people you share this planet with.

> In the end, wellness gives us the chance to live fully—and to make that life one worth living, right up to the very last day.

Dr. Sierra's Magnetic Therapy Protocol

With over four decades of experience in this field, I've developed a system that allows you to combine static magnets, both physiologically and anatomically, with PEMF therapy for personal use. The benefits often become noticeable with consistent application, as magnets help relieve pain and discomfort, reduce inflammation, and improve circulation.

It's well known that magnetic fields interact with magnetic substances such as iron, which is why hemoglobin in the blood becomes more active under magnetic influence. When magnetic energy is applied through either static magnets or PEMF therapy, lymphatic circulation is also stimulated.

My experience leads me to conclude that static magnetic therapy and PEMF energy reactivate what I call our "inner power": our natural ability to resist illness and speed up recovery from fatigue and disease.

Magnetic waves can pass through solid materials, so you don't need to undress or remove your shoes during therapy. Just be sure to take off your watch, as magnetic waves may interfere with its function.

Application

You can use this therapy with a PEMF device of any size, whether it includes a single copper coil or up to eight coils embedded in a cushion. If you don't own a PEMF device, following the instructions for applying static magnets will still provide excellent results.

Place the magnets with the negative north pole facing the skin. Use the following ceramic permanent magnets:

- **N-2**: 4" x 6" x ½"
- **N-1**: 2" x 6" x ½"
- **N-3**: 2" x 3" x ½"
- **Domino magnet**: 1" x 2" x ½"

All are strong and effective.

If you're combining this with electromagnetic therapy, simply position the PEMF applicator over the magnets. Be sure to turn on the machine so the entire body is exposed to the field—you'll feel the effect right away.

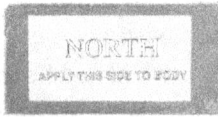

Domino - 1" x 2"

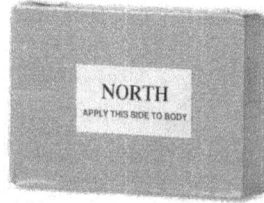

N-3 - 2" x 3"

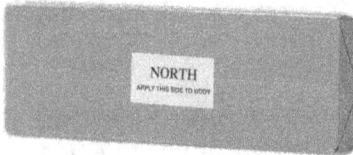

N-1 – 2" x 6"

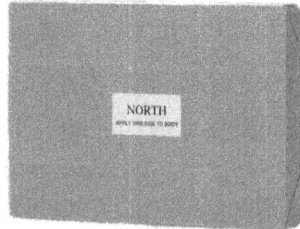

N-2 – 4" x 6"

Start your treatments with twenty-minute intervals (unless a different duration has been specifically recommended). Gradually increase to thirty or forty minutes as your body adjusts to the magnetic waves.

When the body is in balance, optimal results are usually achieved within sessions of twenty to thirty minutes.

You can repeat treatments three to four times per day, and gradually reduce to twice a day, or even once daily, if the pain is no longer intense.

A minimum of two magnets should always be used together. You may use four N magnets at once, plus magnetic hand cylinders. The magnetic energy from each device flows through the body without canceling out other fields. I recommend using at least two magnets for conditions such as neuralgia, rheumatism, diabetes, or any other chronic illness.

For therapeutic purposes, static magnets should typically have a strength between 700 and 3,500 gauss.

General Use For Muscle Aches And Pains

Foot soles, ankles, knees, thighs, hips, buttocks, palms, arms, back and shoulders: 20 to 30 minutes

Head: 10 to 15 minutes

General aches, pains and discomfort to affected areas: 20 to 30 minutes

Magnetic therapy is generally very safe, effective, and free of side effects for most people. You can feel confident using multiple magnets or extending the duration of your sessions, as the body is intelligent enough to absorb only what it needs.

However, there are a few precautions to keep in mind. Avoid PEMF therapy if you have a fever higher than 100°F. The magnetic field stimulates blood circulation, which may cause the fever to rise. Do not use magnetic therapy in cases of active bleeding, whether internal or external. This includes during menstrual periods. Magnetic therapy is not recommended during the last three months of pregnancy. If you have active infections, ulcers, or cancer, it's important to consult a qualified health professional before beginning therapy.

How to Apply Static Magnets

Magnet Positioning

The treatment diagram includes specific symbols to help guide magnet placement:

- **A:** Frontal abdominal and thoracic area

- **B:** Full back

- **S:** Legs

- **Numbers:** Indicate specific contact points according to the diagram

- **Spot:** Refers to a targeted area, chosen based on your condition or the area affected

Basic Treatment

To enhance the body's natural healing power at the most essential points, place domino-type magnets, N-1, N-2, or N-3, with the North pole (negative) touching the skin at the most essential points: 3, 6, 4, 11, and "S". For more specific details regarding a particular problem or condition, please refer to the *Therapeutic Guide* on page 113.

Because the autonomic nervous system begins in the hands and feet, the basic treatment focuses on the most essential points: point 3 (below the navel), 6 (pit of the stomach, solar plexus), 4 (both hands), 11 (mid-back), and the letter "S" (the legs), in order to enhance the body's natural healing power.

When preparing for treatment, you'll combine this information with the specific information for your condition found in the *Therapeutic Guide*. In this way, you combine static and electrical frequencies to achieve better results in your treatment.

If your PEMF device already includes suggested placement positions, you can use those and place the static magnets at the indicated points beneath your PEMF unit. If you are doing your therapy using only static magnets, remember to leave them in place for a longer period of time.

Digestive System

Stomach problems	A	17	S
Diarrhea/constipation	14	5	18
Dyspepsia/gas	6	11	17

Circulatory System

Hypertension	11	16	S
Arteriosclerosis, stroke	7	B	S
Anemia	11	16	S
Low blood pressure	16	B	S

Musculoskeletal System

Arthritis/Rheumatism	Spot	A	S
Spinal herniation	11	B	Spot
Shoulder spasm	4	AB	S

Nervous System

Neuralgia	Spot	B	S	
Facial paralysis	Spot	16	B	
Neuralgia in arm	4	10	12	17
Intercostal neuralgia	Spot	B	S	
Sciatica	13	B	S	
Insomnia, anxiety	16	B	19	
Headache/migraine	19	6	16	

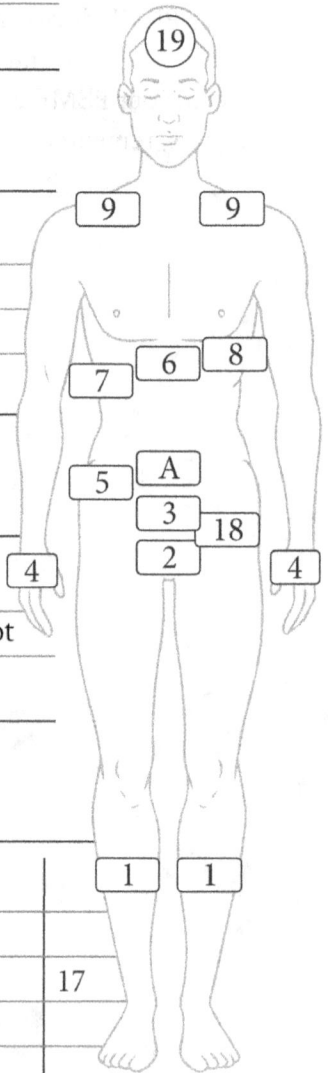

MAGNET POSITIONS

Respiratory System

Asthma	4	9	15	S
Flu, Bronchitis	Spot	B	16	

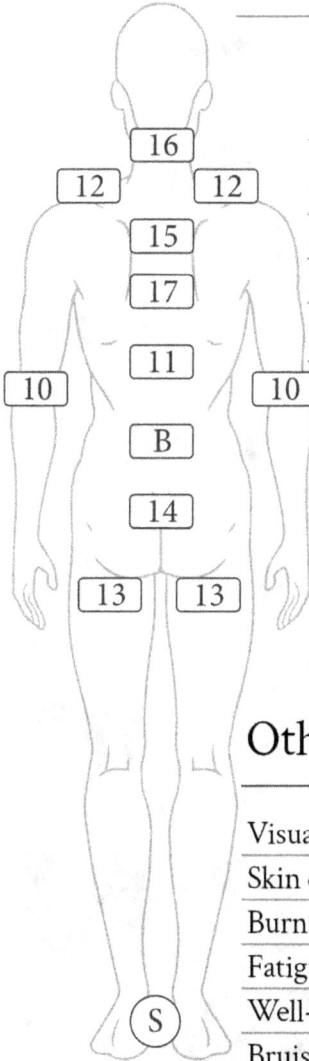

Reproductive System

Cold constitution	1	B	S
Menstrual irregularity	14	A	S
Prostatitis/urethritis	2	14	S
Impotence	Spot	14	S

Urinary System

Kidney	1	B	S
Bladder	2	B	S
Incontinence	2	14	S

Others

Visual fatigue	Spot	4	16	
Skin diseases	Spot	4	16	
Burns	Spot	4	16	
Fatigue/exhaustion	4	A	B	S
Well-being	4	A	B	S
Bruises	Spot			
Toothache	Spot			
Hemorrhoids	Spot			

MAGNET POSITIONS

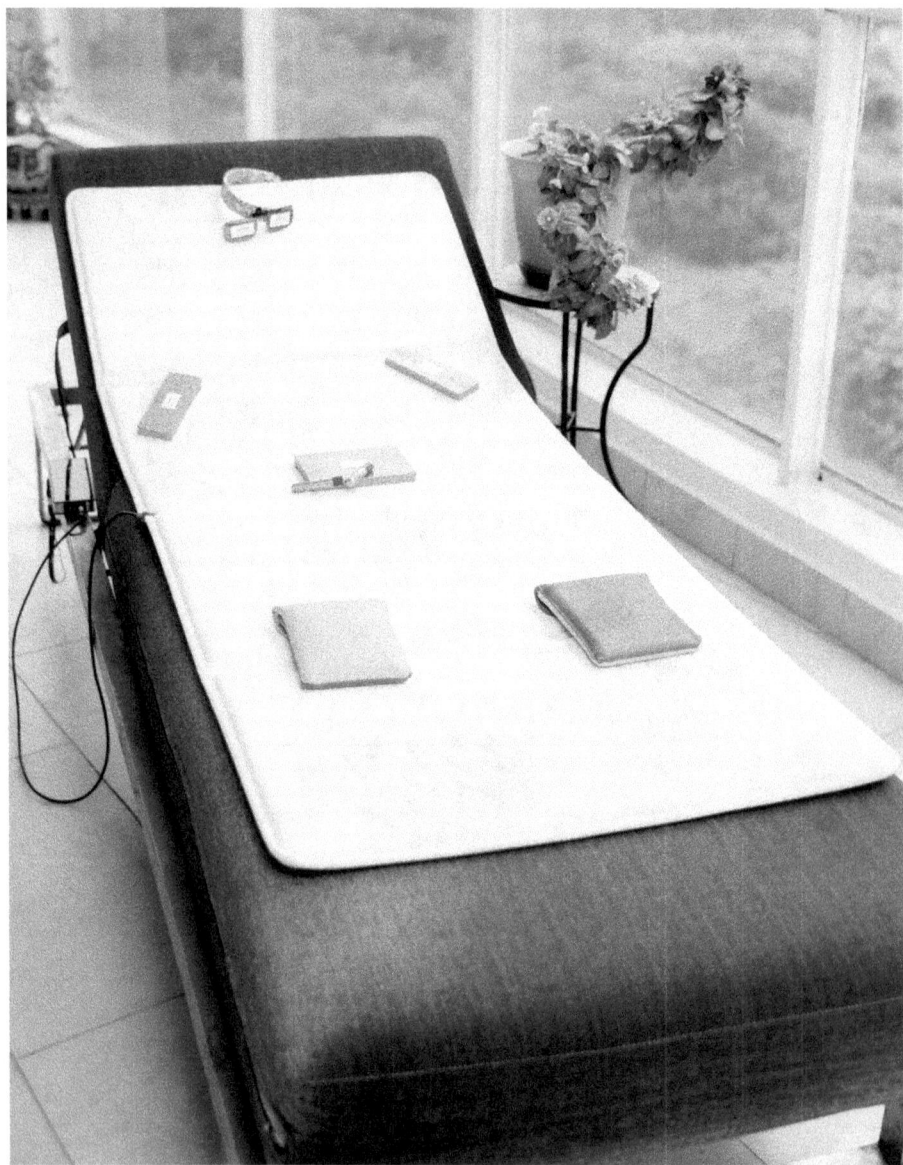

Common Configurations to Use with PEMF Therapy

Musculoskeletal System

Situation	Time	Suggested Frequency
General morning or early morning conditions	8 to 10 minutes	12 to 22 Hz
Night in general (better rest)	8 to 10 minutes	2 or 3 Hz
Dislocations and sprains	20 to 30 minutes	10 Hz
Fibromyalgia	20 minutes	8 to 11 Hz or 15 to 18 Hz
Fractures	20 minutes	10 to 20 Hz
Paralyzed shoulder	20 to 30 minutes	7 or 8 Hz
Herniated disc	20 to 30 minutes	16 to 20 or 30 Hz
Gout	20 minutes	8, 14, 20 or 30 Hz
Inflammation due to injury	20 minutes	8, 14, or 20 Hz
Ligament injuries	20 minutes	10 to 15 Hz
Lumbago	15 minutes	10 to 20 Hz
Muscle spasms	20 minutes	30 to 60 Hz
Musculoskeletal pain	20 minutes	10 Hz
Osteonecrosis/osteochondrosis	20 to 30 minutes	10, 19 or 20 Hz
Osteoporosis	20 minutes	8, 9, 10, 15 or 19 Hz up to 66 Hz
Osteoarthritis	20 minutes	8 to 12 or 18 Hz
Periostitis	20 minutes	6 Hz
Pseudarthrosis (non-union)	20 to 30 minutes	10 to 20 Hz
Rheumatoid arthritis	20 minutes	10 to 20 Hz
Sciatica	20 minutes	16 to 20 Hz
Spinal cord injury	15 minutes	12 to 22 Hz
Overexertion	15 to 20 minutes	11 to 15 Hz
Tendonitis	10 minutes	8 Hz
Tennis elbow (lateral epicondylitis)	10 minutes	8 Hz

Circulatory System

Situation	Time	Frequency
Angina pectoris	20 to 30 minutes	2 to 8 Hz
Arteriosclerosis	15 minutes	7 to 10 Hz
Arrhythmia	20 to 30 minutes	7 to 8 Hz
Bradycardia	20 minutes	8 to 11 Hz
Circulatory dysfunction	15 minutes	7 to 10 Hz
Hearing loss	20 minutes	1 to 5 Hz
Hypertension	20 to 30 minutes (40 Chronic case)	1 to 5 Hz
Heart attack	20 minutes	1 to 5 Hz
Lymphatic disorders	20 to 30 minutes	12 to 22 Hz
Poor blood supply (diabetic foot, ulcer)	20 minutes	2 to 6 or 20 Hz
Raynaud's syndrome	20 minutes	8 to 15 Hz
Stroke	15 minutes	4 to 12 Hz
Tachycardia	20 minutes	1 to 5 Hz

Digestive System

Situation	Time	Frequency
Crohn's disease	20 to 30 minutes	8 to 22 Hz
Dental and oral diseases	30 minutes	30 Hz
Diabetes mellitus	15 to 20 minutes	2 to 6 Hz o 12 to 22 Hz
Inflammation of the liver, pancreas or colon	20 to 30 minutes	12 to 22 Hz
Hepatitis	20 to 30 minutes	12 to 22 Hz
Metabolic disorders	20 minutes	8 to 11 Hz
Stomach ulcer/duodenal ulcer (no hemorrhage)	12 minutes	10 to 20 Hz
Stomachaches	12 minutes	10 Hz

Nervous System/Neurological Condition

Situation	Time	Frequency
Alzheimer's disease	20 to 30 minutes	2 to 8 Hz
Carpal tunnel syndrome	10 minutes	6 to 20 Hz
Depression	10 minutes	3 to 20 Hz
Early-onset dementia	20 to 30 minutes	12 to 22 Hz
Headaches	15 minutes	3 to 6 or 10 Hz
Hyperactivity	10 minutes	8 to 11 Hz
Migraines	20 minutes	8 to 11 Hz
Multiple sclerosis	20 to 30 minutes	5, 13 or 20 Hz
Nerve pain	10 minutes	6 Hz
Panic attacks	20 minutes	15 to 26 Hz
Parkinson's disease	20 to 30 minutes	20 Hz
Sensitivity to weather fronts	10 minutes	11 to 15 Hz
Sleep disorders/insomnia	10 to 20 minutes	1 to 5 Hz
Stress	15 minutes	3 to 5 Hz
Tinnitus	20 minutes	10 Hz

Respiratory System

Situation	Time	Frequency
Allergies	10 minutes	5 to 10 Hz
Asthma	20 minutes	7 to 10 Hz or 12 to 15 Hz
Bronchitis	12 minutes	4 to 12 Hz
Hay fever	20 to 30 minutes	12 to 22 Hz
Pneumonia, respiratory diseases	20 to 30 minutes	12 to 22 Hz
Tuberculosis (Tb)	12 minutes	4 Hz

Others

Situation	Time	Frequency
Chronic blepharitis	20 to 30 minutes	1 or 2 Hz
Chronic fatigue	20 to 30 minutes	12 to 22 Hz
Chronic pelvic pain	20 minutes	5 to 7 Hz
Cystitis	20 minutes	5 to 8 Hz
Detoxification	20 minutes	8 to 11 Hz
Erectile dysfunction	20 minutes	6 Hz
Glaucoma, atrophy of the optic nerve	20 to 30 minutes	12 to 22 Hz
Gynecological inflammation	20 minutes	8 to 11 Hz
Menstrual cramps	20 minutes	5 to 7 Hz
Prostatitis	10 to 15 minutes	2 to 8 Hz
Psoriasis	20 to 30 minutes	12 to 22 Hz
Rest and relaxation	20 minutes	8 to 11 Hz
Revitalize	20 minutes	12 to 22 Hz
Strengthening immunity	20 minutes	8 to 11 Hz
Systemic Lupus Erythematosus (SLE)	20 minutes	12 to 22 Hz
Bruises	15 minutes	10 Hz
Burns	20 minutes	8 to 11 Hz
Pain associated with wound healing	15 minutes	11 to 15 or 17 Hz
Phantom pain	15 minutes	16 to 19 Hz
Wound healing	15 minutes	1 to 5 Hz

Therapeutic Guide

These protocols are based on Irma Sierra's personal experience and long-standing practice with magnetic therapy.

1. **Abscesses:** Apply the negative north pole of the magnet directly to the affected area for fifteen minutes, three to four times a day. Polarize water with the negative north pole and use it to clean the area.

2. **Acidity/Low Alkalinity:** Locate the focal point of pain and apply the negative north pole there. Drink water magnetized with the negative north pole. PEMF therapy is also recommended.

3. **Acne:** Apply any magnet to the affected area for thirty minutes. Magnetize astringent with a domino magnet and apply it with a cotton pad three times a day. For severe acne, use the face mask, which provides full-face coverage with negative north pole energy. Also drink plenty of water magnetized with the negative north pole, and wash affected areas with it. Consider evaluating your diet, especially for possible dairy allergies.

4. **Addiction:** Increase daily use of negative north pole magnets to calm the hyperactivity caused by positive south magnetic stimulation and to restore balance in the brain and body. Sleep with the magnets and follow your nightly routine. Use ceramic magnets over the liver, pancreas, diaphragm, or anywhere you feel discomfort. To soothe emotional stress during withdrawal, apply two domino magnets on the temples, just above and in front of the ears. The face mask can also help increase exposure to negative magnetic energy.

5. **Aging:** Magnets activate life-promoting enzyme activity which, in turn, promotes normal cell division. This encourages the organism to be healthy and to even slow down the aging process. To balance the energy within all the glands and organs in the body I suggest applying magnetic fields all around the body. Sleeping on top of magnets in bed is a great way to achieve that. Another good habit you can adopt to assist your body is consuming more polarized water. You can also strengthen the injured or weak areas of the body by applying magnets to these areas.

6. **Alcoholism:** Apply the negative north pole over the liver, pancreas, diaphragm, and the nape of the neck (base of the skull) to ease withdrawal symptoms. Drink water magnetized with the negative north pole.

7. **Allergies:** Allergic reactions can affect many systems: spleen, thymus, lymph nodes, sinuses, throat, lungs, gastrointestinal tract, skin, eyes, and brain. Negative magnetic energy helps normalize immune responses, reduce inflammation, and soothe symptoms.

    a) **Skin Allergies:** Apply a magnet over the affected area. If you're using a body lotion, store the lotion on top of the negative north pole when not in use.

    b) **Eye Allergies**: Use Dr. Sierra's eye shields with eyes closed for fifteen to thirty minutes.

    c) **General Allergies**: Apply the N-2 magnet twice daily to the spleen, and the N-1 magnet to the thymus. Drink plenty of magnetized water.

8. **Amenorrhea (Scarce or Absent Menstruation):** Apply the negative north pole to the pelvic zone to reduce discomfort. For regulation, apply the positive south pole to the same area for thirty to sixty minutes, twice a day. Follow up with the negative north pole to regain energetic balance. Nutritional support with vitamins B, C, and D is also recommended.

9. **Amputations:** Many people with amputations experience phantom limb pain, often linked to vascular issues.

Research suggests magnets can help improve blood flow to the residual limb and reduce or eliminate phantom pain (Casale et al., 2009; Pasek et al., 2012).

10. **Anemia:** Wear a magnetic bracelet, regardless of polarity, to support iron levels. Drink water magnetized with both north and south poles, ideally using the magnetic pen for best results.

11. **Angina:** Must be diagnosed and monitored by a health professional. Carry a small negative north pole magnet over the heart (in a shirt pocket or attached to clothing). Discontinue use immediately if discomfort occurs. Drink water magnetized with the negative north pole. Important: Do not use if you have a pacemaker.

12. **Anorexia:** Apply the positive south pole of an N-1 magnet to the upper abdomen or thoracic spine area (T10 & T11) near the navel for thirty minutes. Then apply the negative north pole for another thirty minutes to re-balance. You may also wear the positive south pole on your left wrist or hold a magnetic cylinder in your left hand. Drink dual-polarity magnetized water using the magnetic pen.

13. **Anxiety:** Place the negative north pole of a domino magnet on the stomach area and another on the lower cervical spine for fifteen to thirty minutes, twice daily or as needed. The neckband is also highly recommended. Drink water magnetized with the negative north pole and wear a negative-polarity magnetic bracelet regularly.

14. **Appendicitis:** Seek emergency medical care immediately. While waiting or if surgery isn't required, apply the negative north pole over the appendix area for forty-five minutes, twice daily. Use the flexible magnetic pad, N-1, or domino magnets in a back support belt, positioned on the right lower abdomen. Drink north polarized water.

15. **Arrhythmia:**Requires professional diagnosis and monitoring. You may place a small negative north pole magnet over the heart

area (shirt pocket or clothing). Discontinue immediately if discomfort occurs. Drink north-polarized water. Important: Do not use if you have a pacemaker.

16.   **Arthritis:** There's a variety of supportive equipment available for all joints of the body. Start with a magnetic bed if you have difficulty moving, or even use a simple magnetic wrist, knee or neck brace. Pain is often linked to inflammation, and applying a magnet directly can help reduce it. If you experience an increase in pain, decrease the treatment time and then gradually increase its use. In some cases of rheumatoid arthritis, fluid accumulation can be found in the joint and the magnet may attract additional fluid thus increasing pain, although this isn't a common occurrence. It's also helpful to move the magnet to different areas of the body. We should all consider wearing at least one magnetic bracelet. Magnetic rings are excellent for treating arthritis localized to the finger. It's also recommended you drink magnetized water. To stop the affliction, you can directly apply the negative north pole of a magnet to the skin, having direct contact with the affected area. Regularly rolling magnetic balls (of both polarities) on the hands or other parts of the body is a very effective treatment for arthritic conditions, especially in the hands and fingers. Placing the negative north pole of a magnet over the inflamed area on a regular basis could be the key to improvement, especially in cases of arthritis in the hands and feet.

17.   **Asthma:** Place a negative north pole magnet over the chest covering the bronchi and on the back at the same level can help with this affliction. Sleeping on a magnetic mattress can also be very beneficial. It may take several days before you can breathe normally again, but the magnets can be worn continuously during this time. Apply the negative north pole to the chest over the sternum, two inches under the clavicles. On the back apply the positive south pole magnet over the T2 and T5 areas. Two domino shaped magnets or small flexible pads are more than enough. On the onset of an acute bronchospasm, remove the negative north pole magnet, then reapply it for fifteen to thirty minutes

after the bronchospasm to help reduce inflammation and swelling. Drink water magnetized with the negative north pole.

18. **Atherosclerosis:** Hardening of the arteries can result in decreased circulation to the brain, heart and extremities. Which is why applying negative magnetic therapy to the blood prevents fatty materials and fatty acids from sticking to the arterial walls, avoiding swelling and the development of plaques inside them. In some cases, magnetic therapy has been successful in reversing the course of this disease. Use magnets such as the N-1 over the navel, flexible pads or back supports for one hour a day. This can increase the negative polarity of the blood vessels. You can also place the N-1 or N-2 magnets on the bifurcation of the aorta, which is to say on the right and left side of the groin area where the leg joins the body. Additionally, wearing magnetic jewelry with a negative north pole on the ankles and wrists magnetizes the blood while you go on with your day. To also benefit your brain, sleep with a magnet under your pillow. I also recommend wearing Dr. Sierra's magnetic neckband, using the memory band or placing the N-1 or N-2 ceramic magnet at the base of the skull. If you don't have a pacemaker, you can place a magnet over your heart, but not for more than 30 minutes at a time. Using soles magnetized with both polarities if there's no pain present, hypertension or varicose veins can improve circulation on the legs. Soles magnetized with the negative north pole will work the same way. Making use of magnets all around the body is the best way to prevent this health problem.

19. **Atrophy:** Sit on top of a magnetic pillow alternating between the negative north pole and positive south pole for eight to ten hours. Make use of magnetic soles too and if possible, hold a cylinder in your hands for fifteen minutes each. When sleeping with magnets in bed I suggest alternating the poles. Have five days of the negative north pole on the upper area and two days with the positive south pole on the upper area. It is important to analyze its strength and adjust the polarity according to its weakness com-

pared to its strength. Use magnetic soles and drink water magnetized with the negative north pole and positive south pole. A practical option is the use of the magnetic pen.

20. **Autoimmune diseases:** Diseases such as rheumatoid arthritis, AIDS, and other autoimmune conditions should be diagnosed by a health professional as early as possible for best results. The incidence of many of these autoimmune diseases has increased due to the decrease of the magnetic field in the body. It's important to take care of your magnetic field and make sure to feed and maintain it through magnetic therapy. Besides using magnets you can make changes in your diet as well to help your body recover. Completely eliminate gluten, reduce your daily stress, increase your water intake and practice relaxation techniques such as yoga, Tai-chi or Qi-Gong. Pulsating electromagnetic therapy treats the affected organ, reduces stress and inflammation within the body, prevents additional damage and stops the progression of autoimmune problems. Autoimmune diseases make you sensitive not only to nutrition, but also to medications and environmental stimuli. Tailor this therapeutic method to your individual needs. Magnetic therapies, both static and pulsed, will help reduce the severity and duration of autoimmune episodes, as well as reduce organ damage.

21. **Back pain:** This pain can be treated effectively through the application of the negative north pole. This is achieved with the magnetic back band. It's important to consider the necessary length so the magnetic energy can travel through the whole body. In some cases adding another pad or an N-1 or N-3 magnet to improve discomfort quicker is needed.

22. **Bacterial, fungal, viral, parasitic infections:** It's important to avoid the use of the positive south pole in these situations. I recommend you wash the infected area with water magnetized with the negative north pole apply this same polarity to the area for an hour, three to four times a day, until the condition improves. I suggest covering this area with gauze before applying the magnet. Drink water magnetized with the negative north

pole, this will help avoid the systematic propagation of the infection. I also suggest you sleep on top of a magnet. Wash your mouth with polarized water to alkalinize the body. For lung infections, apply the ceramic N-1 or N-2 magnets to the affected lung area for at least three hours a day or as long as possible. For urinary bladder and kidney infections, you can apply magnets to the affected areas for up to two or three days after the symptoms disappear. Seek medical attention if the symptoms do not improve.

23. **Bell's palsy:** Apply the negative north pole to the affected side of the face first, and then apply the positive south pole to the facial muscles for thirty minutes. Also apply the same sequence to the seventh cranial nerve behind the ear. Use a negative north pole face mask for thirty to sixty minutes, and alternate placements between the cheek, lower jaw, and facial muscles. Supplement treatment with vitamin B-12 and herbal remedies for pain and inflammation.

24. **Bladder problems:** Apply the negative north pole directly to the lower abdomen. This is helpful in cases of infection, weakness, or bladder distention. Apply twice a day for at least thirty minutes. If the bladder is extremely weak but not infected, you may also use the positive south pole to help strengthen it. Alternate between poles at different times of the day but never use both simultaneously. I also suggest magnetic soles with both polarities and plenty of polarized water. The magnetic pencil works well for this purpose.

25. **Bleeding/hemorrhage:** Sitting on a negative north pole magnet can help reduce or stop hemorrhaging, including rectal bleeding and heavy menstruation. Sit for thirty to forty minutes in the morning and evening. Recovery time depends on your specific symptoms. Magnetic therapy has proven effective in stopping bleeding caused by weak tissue. Drink plenty of polarized water.

26. **Blepharitis/conjunctivitis:** To treat swollen eyelids apply Dr. Sierra's magnetic eye mask for fifteen to thirty minutes in the morning and at night. Apply it a third time during the day if

you deem it necessary. If you don't have these items available, you can apply negative north pole magnets to the area around your eyes for fifteen minutes every two to three hours. You must wash your eyes with water magnetized with the negative north pole and apply eye cream that's also been magnetized by the same pole every two to three hours.

27. **Blood clots:** Apply a negative north pole magnet directly over the blood clot. This tends to slowly reduce the clot. Use the domino shaped magnet, a magnetic point of a loose leg wrap. You don't have to apply it with too much strength on top or around the area. The blood clot should start dissolving.

28. **Bones and joints:** If the person isn't experiencing muscle weakness or stiffness and can stand and even walk short distances, the recommendation is to apply the negative north pole. For each joint of the body there is a specific magnet, and if you follow the specifications of this guide, you can treat them all. Magnetic therapy is highly effective and it can be combined with other forms of treatment such as chiropractics, as the application of the magnet helps retain the "adjustment" for longer periods of time. By applying magnets to bones, muscles or joints (tendons, ligaments or cartilage) you encourage strengthening and bone and tissue repair to the point of regeneration. That is with constant daily application, even while sleeping, and without causing discomfort. Patience is essential, as results may take months or even years, depending on how long you've experienced the problems over time.

29. **Breasts:** Apply small negative north pole magnets (can be domino-sized) to the sides of the breasts. For sensitivity, attach these magnets to a bra. For fissures from breastfeeding, place the magnets directly over the affected area. Use static and pulsed therapy (magnets will not damage implants). Therapy helps reduce swelling, pain, and excessive scarring.

30. **Bronchitis:** Place the negative north pole against the nose, then the throat and then the lungs for eight minutes in each location. Apply with frequency depending on the pain level.

31. **Bulging or herniated discs:** Disc problems are a common concern in the chiropractic field. Try to always have a magnetic back support and always wear the flexible pad. It complements any therapy. If the pain radiates down the legs, it is advisable to use magnetic insoles. Sleeping on a magnetic cushion or mattress can be beneficial. You can also modify a seat cushion with magnets so that you can sit on it. It's important to take supplements and hydrate the affected area. Drink plenty of magnetized water to keep the body in optimal condition.

32. **Burns:** Magnets can speed up the healing of most first-degree burns. For minor burns, apply magnets directly over the area. For more severe burns, magnetic therapy can help reduce the need for painkillers. Apply the negative north pole as soon as possible, before blisters form, for thirty to forty minutes. Use domino-shaped or N-1 magnets depending on the burn size. You can also soak gauze in polarized water or magnetized aloe juice and place it over the skin to accelerate healing. Once the burn begins to heal and shows no signs of infection, use the positive south pole to encourage new tissue growth. Repeat as needed until the burn is fully healed.

33. **Bursitis:** A very painful swelling that is often produced in the shoulder or hip joint. Apply three or four magnetic spots around the joint for twenty four hour therapy. You can attach them with a bandage that can last from three to five days. They can be used in the shower, that way you don't have to remove and reapply them often. Magnets are reusable. Note: While feeling relief may take weeks, you will have your mobility back before then. In the meantime, you should rest and avoid strenuous activities.

34. **Cancer:** N-1 or N-2 are designed with the negative north pole on one side and the positive south pole on the other. They have over 3,000 gauss and they can be kept towards the body for long periods of time. Roy Davis' research (see letters in the chapter on The Story of Sierra and Davis) recommends applying them for forty five minutes three times a day for three weeks on the cancerous area. The treatment time is to be determined depending

on the magnitude of it. For example, if it's breast cancer, the domino sized negative north pole magnet is placed inside the bra or held in place with adhesive tape. On two occasions, my husband and I have been speakers, following in Ralph's footsteps, at the Cancer Control Society where we talked about how essential the negative north pole is to treating those cancer cells, and the importance of attacking them as early as possible to give hope of controlling their growth. An important observation is that we advise every patient we receive who is undergoing chemotherapy treatment to take the N-1 magnet with them and apply it to their stomach while receiving this therapy. We do this to reduce or even avoid any symptoms that come from being exposed to these harmful chemicals on a daily basis. You can find our lecture in the references section (Power in a Magnet Part 1. Aug 2017, n.d.).

35. **Candidiasis:** You should treat this condition as you would an infection. Sit on an N-1 negative north pole magnetic chair or cushion for one hour, two to three times a day to help alleviate symptoms. If you keep using magnets, you will feel and experience less recurrence. They could even disappear completely.

36. **Carotid Arteries:** Use Dr. Sierra's neckband, placing two domino magnets with the north pole facing inwards, applied to one side of the throat.

37. **Carpal Tunnel Syndrome (CTS):** For CTS, position magnets on the front and back of the wrist. Relief can often be achieved with a negative north pole magnetic wrist brace. Wearing a magnetic bracelet regularly has also proven helpful for many people. Do not delay treatment. Addressing the issue early increases the chances of long-term improvement.

38. **Cataracts:** The best way to use Dr. Sierra's magnetic glasses is to wear them for ten to fifteen minutes once or twice a day. Keep a day of rest where you don't use them. This practice has proven to be more effective in general. In more severe cases increase the session to thirty minutes. Be seated or lying down when wearing the magnetic glasses. Take advantage of the moment and rest,

relax and even meditate. Throughout Dr. Sierra's research, which lasted about eleven years, compared to my forty years of research and the years of selling these magnetic glasses, I've personally seen improvements in about 80% of the cases, while only 20% show no apparent improvement. Research also revealed that intraocular pressure has decrease in glaucoma cases. It can take days or up to months to see results, but if you're consistent, you'll experience relief.

39. **Cellulite/fat deposits:** Energy from the north negative pole is alkaline and neutralizes the acid in adipose tissue which dissolves the fatty substance. Apply the magnets directly to the fatty tissues located on the thighs, buttocks and upper arms while you sleep to dissolve cellulite. Drink water magnetized with the negative north pole, change your diet, add exercise and massages to your routine. You will see results, just not as soon as you'd like. Good and effective processes take time!

40. **Cervicitis:** Apply a negative north pole magnet to the pubic bone. Then sit over a negative north pole magnet for forty minutes two to three times a day. Drink water magnetized with the negative north pole.

41. **Chronic Fatigue Syndrome (CFS)/Myalgic Encephalomyelitis:** To be diagnosed with CFS, a person must experience persistent fatigue along with other symptoms for at least six months. Usual symptoms include lack of energy, widespread pain, frequent headaches, and dizziness, many of which overlap with magnetic field deficiency syndrome. External magnetic therapy helps by re-balancing the body's energy. I recommend wearing magnetic jewelry, using magnetic pads, shoe insoles, and sleeping on magnetic cushions. Drink polarized water daily. Use a magnetic massager or cylinder on reflexology points and over affected areas for fifteen seconds to fifteen minutes to increase energy. See also the section on autoimmune conditions, as recent studies suggest that immune dysfunction may be involved (Sotzny et al., 2018).

42. **Circulatory problems:** You can wear magnetic bands along your forearms and sleep on a magnetic pad at night.

Negative magnetic energy helps normalize the acid-alkaline pH balance of elements like cholesterol and triglycerides, which tend to accumulate inside arterial walls. When applying negative north pole energy, the magnetic waves penetrate tissue and create secondary electrical currents. These currents generate heat, which affects the body's cellular electrons. This activates hemoglobin and accelerates blood flow, which can gradually reduce calcium and cholesterol deposits. Since fat tissue is acidic, the alkalizing effect of the negative north pole also helps neutralize and dissolve fat. Keep in mind this is a gradual process.

43. **Colds, congestion:** Apply the negative north pole to the nose area, followed by the throat and the chest (above the lungs), for seven to eight minutes each. This often helps relieve cold symptoms. Wear magnetic bands around your neck, use negative north pole magnetic jewelry, and drink polarized water and liquids to support your immune system. If you have congestion but no infection, apply the positive south pole to the lungs. For infections, inflammation, or pus, use the negative north pole to help control bacterial development. Although magnets won't eliminate an infection, they can help halt its progression so your body can recover naturally.

44. **Constipation or diarrhea:** Treating the intestinal tract involves treating all the organs located in the abdomen. Negative north pole magnetic therapy should be applied over the liver, gallbladder and colon. Sleeping with an N-2 magnet under your back at night helps retain liquid in the feces, and the magnetic back belt will provide additional benefits. To treat diarrhea, I recommend first applying the positive south pole to the lower left abdominal region followed by the negative north pole. For both intestinal problems I recommend drinking water magnetized with the negative north pole. PEMF therapy may be beneficial for this condition as well.

45. **Cystitis:** I recommend drinking water magnetized with the negative north pole and sitting on an N-1 negative north pole pillow or magnetic cushion for a minimum of three hours, for at least

thirty minutes per session. You can also use ceramic magnets over the kidneys, bladder and ureters for one to three hours daily or continuously until symptoms improve and disappear. You can add a magnetic belt for the back but placing it over the abdomen.

46. **Dandruff:** Magnetize your hair care products with the negative north pole and drink water magnetized with the negative north pole.

47. **Depression:** Sleep with a magnet under the pillow or on a magnetic bed. Wearing magnetic jewelry on the left hand can help if the depression comes with anxiety. When magnets are placed around the head, they help uplift the mood and promote relaxation. Drinking water magnetized with the negative north pole will also be helpful. Transcranial PEMF therapy to treat depression is FDA-approved.

48. **Dermatitis:** Since magnets reduce any sort of swelling, you can place them in any area where the skin is inflamed, red or swelled. Inflamed, reddened and itchy skin see favorable results with this treatment.

49. **Diabetes:** Apply the positive south pole of a domino shaped magnet to the upper left part of the abdomen, 2" directly under the nipple for thirty minutes twice a day. This helps reduce the glucose levels in the blood. I suggest monitoring your sugar levels in case you need to reduce the intensity of the magnetic therapy to avoid a low blood sugar episode. Drink water magnetized with the negative north pole.

50. **Diverticulitis:** To relieve pain apply the negative north pole of the magnet to the affected area. You can wear a magnetic band on your back throughout the day and you can also sleep with it facing your abdomen, specifically towards the north. It's important to drink six to eight cups of water magnetized with the negative north pole a day. In case of constipation, place the positive south pole on the lower left side of the abdomen for thirty minutes and then remove it. Balance is restored when using the negative north pole after using the positive south pole of the

magnet. I also recommend the use of a negative north pole magnetic pad.

51. **Dizziness:** For motion sickness on land, sea, or air, magnetized wristbands targeting acupuncture points can be effective. Magnets may also be placed under the ears or on the back of the head. Drink plenty of polarized water before, during, and after exposure to the motion that caused the dizziness.

52. **Down syndrome:** Many have asked whether children with Down syndrome can use magnets, and the answer is yes. My brother Marcel, who had Down syndrome, was a gifted dancer and athlete. He used magnets whenever he felt discomfort. In our home, we only drank water magnetized by placing a jar over a 5" round ceramic magnet with the negative north pole facing up. Although Down syndrome is a genetic condition, individuals with it can experience various neurological symptoms. Magnetic therapy is safe, non-invasive, and suitable for children three years of age and older.

53. **Earache:** Position a domino shaped magnet over the affected ear and sleep on that side with the ear to the pillow. Make sure the magnet stays under the ear. You can also place magnets on the throat, neck and nape of the neck. Leave them on until you feel relief. In some cases, it's possible for pain to increase drastically before it disappears completely. Apply a negative north pole magnet over each ear for twenty to thirty minutes, two to three times a day.

54. **Eczema:** Apply the negative north pole of the magnet to the affected area for three hours. Drink and wash the area with water magnetized with the negative north pole.

55. **Edema:** If you're suffering from edema you should consider the possibility that you may have an underlying disease. It's imperative that you are evaluated by a health professional and treated with magnetic therapy. Conditions such as swelling on the arms or legs caused by reduced blood or a reduction on the lymphatic return flow requires special attention. Place the magnets directly

over the affected area. If the swelling is associated with scar tissue or with a lesion near an obstruction place ceramic magnets directly over the obstruction to encourage resolution. For edema on the ankles, besides elevating your legs, use negative north pole ankle braces and be sure to hydrate with polarized water.

56. **Emotional disorders:** The central nervous system (CNS) plays a key role in regulating our emotions. Maintaining a balance between stimulating and calming signals, represented by the magnetic polarities, is essential. As mentioned earlier, the brain responds positively to negative magnetic energy. Apply the negative north pole to the forehead and the occipital region (base of the skull) for fifteen to thirty minutes. In cases of schizophrenia, I recommend applying the negative north pole to both temporal bones. A negative north pole magnetic headband can promote a calming effect. Avoid applying positive south pole energy to the brain, as negative energy helps calm excessive neural activity and hormone production. Though it may seem unusual, sitting on a magnetic cushion or placing N-1 magnets beneath you can also provide significant emotional relief.

57. **Emotional or physical stress/strain:** I suggest you seek relaxation by lying on top of a magnetic pillow to calm the nervous system and soothe your emotional state, as well as provide the body with a full therapy. Wearing magnetic jewelry based on negative north pole energy can be useful to face daily challenges.

58. **Emphysema:** In cases of emphysema, the lungs tend to close, limiting the absorption and use of air. There's a state of congestion that restricts breathing. It's crucial to open these pulmonary structures, and the use of the north negative pole followed by the use of positive south energy can help expand and strengthen the tissue. I recommend you apply each pole for twenty five minutes twice a day. Important note! Do not use or apply magnets in the thoracic area if you have a defibrillator or a pacemaker.

59. **Epilepsy:** It's fundamental that you are diagnosed by a specialist before even considering magnetic therapy to treat epilepsy.

Place the negative north pole under your head. You can place it under the pillow every night or place the magnetic wrap on top of the head. This will normalize brain's pH level and bring it to an alkaline state, as well as provide oxygen to the brain cells. That same energy will attack any hidden or unseen infection. Drink water magnetized with the negative north pole and positive south pole.

60. **Facial paralysis:** Use the magnetic face mask to help tone facial muscles. Apply the negative north pole with a domino magnet to tighten the muscle and the positive south pole to help it relax.

61. **Female disorders:**

   a) **Conception aid:** Sit on a positive south pole magnet for thirty minutes twice daily, preferably in the morning and evening. Ensure there is no infection present before beginning this practice. This application helps strengthen the muscles and tissues in the reproductive area, supporting conception. Discontinue once pregnancy is achieved.

   b) **Endometriosis:** Magnetic therapy can be both relieving and beneficial, although results may take several months of consistent use. In our practice, we have seen positive outcomes using a 2,500-gauss magnet placed over the lower abdomen for six to twelve hours daily.

   c) **Fibroids:** Apply a negative north pole magnet over the lower abdominal region, even in cases where fibroids are large enough to potentially require surgery. This therapy may help reduce their size and impact while also relieving pain.

   d) **Hemorrhages:** Sit on a negative north pole magnet for thirty minutes once or twice daily to help stop excessive bleeding. This polarity also helps regulate excessive fluid production.

e) **Hot flashes:** Provided there are no uterine or ovarian cysts present, you can apply a flexible positive south pole magnetic pad over the ovaries for thirty minutes to help stimulate hormone production. Follow by switching to the negative north pole for the rest of the day or night.

f) **Leucorrhea (excessive vaginal discharge):** Place the negative north pole magnet over the perineum, pubic area, ovaries, and uterus for at least three hours a day. If constipation is present, apply the positive south pole to the lower abdomen for ten to fifteen minutes, then immediately switch to the negative north pole. Drink water magnetized with both poles and bathe in water magnetized with the negative north pole. Consult a specialist if symptoms persist beyond three to five days.

g) **Menopausal discomfort:** Use negative north pole magnets or a magnetic pillow to ease menopausal symptoms. You may also apply the negative north pole magnet to the left palm and under the right foot, while placing the positive south pole magnet on the right palm and under the left foot for ten minutes in the morning. Drink water magnetized with the negative north pole and sleep on a magnetic pillow.

h) **Menstrual discomfort and pain:** Place the negative north pole magnet over the uterus for at least thirty minutes daily for seven to ten days. You can alternate between the negative north and positive south poles for the same time. Drink water magnetized with the negative north pole. You may also apply the negative north pole magnet to the left palm and under the right foot, while placing the positive south pole magnet on the right palm and under the left foot for ten minutes in the morning. When placed over the lower abdomen, a magnetic cushion or wrap helps relieve inflammation and pain associated with menstruation.

i) **Menstrual irregularity:** Use the same technique described above. Wearing a magnetic wrap on the forehead may support nervous system regulation.

j) **Ovarian or uterine cysts:** Always obtain a medical diagnosis. Magnetic therapy may be used to complement conventional treatments. Place a negative north pole magnet continuously over the ovaries and drink water magnetized with the negative north pole.

k) **PMS (premenstrual syndrome):** Apply flexible pads, domino-shaped magnets, or a magnetic belt below the navel. Sleeping on a magnetic bed can help if symptoms are widespread. For localized symptoms, apply magnets directly to the area of discomfort.

l) **Pregnancy:** While no specific studies confirm the effects of magnetic therapy during pregnancy, avoid applying magnets directly to the abdomen. You may, however, use magnetic jewelry, point magnets, or supports for the neck, legs, arms, or wrists, as these do not penetrate deeply. For low back pain, 800-gauss magnetic points are considered safe when used on the lumbar or sacroiliac joints.

m) **Sex:** If your libido has decreased, sitting on a positive south pole magnet for thirty minutes before bedtime may help. This stimulates nerve activity and strengthens the reproductive organs.

n) **Vaginal problems or infections:** Sit on a negative north pole magnet for one to two hours, two to three times per day. Also, apply the negative north pole over the uterus and pelvic region. Bathe with water magnetized with the negative north pole and drink water of the same polarity.

62. **Fever:** Fever is a symptom of an infection. Drink water magnetized with the negative north pole and ice your head.

63. **Fibromyalgia:** To treat inflammation, I recommend using all negative north pole magnets. This includes pillows, seat cushions,

wraps, braces, bands or magnetic spots. Using negative north pole magnets on pillows or under it can alleviate discomfort associated with depression, anxiety, poor memory or concentration, and insomnia. In addition, although it's uncomfortable initially, if you persevere, chiropractic treatment is extremely beneficial. In a few weeks after continuous treatment you'll start feeling the positive changes. It's of utmost importance that you keep hydrated with polarized water. You can also place magnets on the areas that hurt during the day to feel relief.

64.   **Foot and leg problems:** Magnetic insoles will help increase circulation and relieve symptoms such as numbness, burning, pain, restlessness, and cramps in the legs. I also recommend sleeping on a magnetic pad.

65.   **Fractured bones:** When a bone breaks, it turns into two different magnets with positive and negative polarities that repel each other. To help the body heal, visit a specialist to get a cast that can hold the bones in place. Place the positive south pole of a magnet, of whatever size necessary depending of the fracture location, over the fracture. The positive south pole softens the zone and releases the calcium from the upper part. Simultaneously, place the surface of the negative north pole of another magnet over the inferior side of the fracture to attract fluids and calcium towards the current position. This way, the negative north pole is helping the calcium redirect to where it needs to go, accelerating the healing process of the bone.

66.   **Gastrointestinal disorders:** To relieve discomfort, apply the negative north pole over the area of concern, such as the gallbladder, stomach, or intestines. For gas or flatulence, often caused by poor digestion or excess stomach acid, improvement has been observed with the application of the positive south pole of the N-1 magnet, or even with magnetic cloths and points. Apply them over the stomach for twenty to thirty minutes once or twice a day. According to Davis and Sierra, the positive south pole can enhance natural stomach acids, helping to relieve digestive discomfort effectively. In some cases, indigestion is due to low

stomach acid levels. For diarrhea and constipation (two different energetic expressions) individual testing is recommended to determine what works best. Generally, applying the negative north pole to the lower abdomen is safe. The positive south pole may help relax the muscles in cases of constipation, while the negative north pole is often more suitable for diarrhea. Place the magnet directly over the navel for thirty minutes per session. Sleeping with a magnetic brace over the abdominal area, with the negative north pole facing the skin, is also beneficial.

67. **Glaucoma:** Hardening of the eyes. Glaucoma causes the internal pressure of the eye to increase due to the trapped fluids. Use the negative north pole eye shields over you eyes for fifteen minutes twice a day. This will also help you reduce pain and pressure.

68. **Goiter:** Place the negative north pole on the palm of your left hand and under the right foot. Place the positive south pole on the palm of your right hand and under the left foot. Do this for ten minutes a day in the morning. You can position the negative north pole of your magnetic collar towards the front of the neck, pointing to the thyroids, for thirty five minutes four to five times a day. Keep hydrated with water magnetized with the negative north pole.

69. **Gout:** This condition pushes the body into an acidic state, so make sure to drink six to eight glasses of water magnetized with the negative north pole, wear magnetic jewelry and apply the magnet directly over the affected joint.

70. **Hair loss:** Stimulating the hair follicles with a magnetic brush is very beneficial for hair growth. Brush with the magnetic brush in the areas where hair loss is more common and you could see some degree of hair recovery. However, the results may vary depend on the underlying cause of the hair loss and how consistently the hair is brushed with the magnetic brush.

71. **Head injuries:** Even mild head injuries can lead to chronic issues like headaches, memory loss, chronic fatigue syndrome, vision problems, and irritability. To help the body correct the

electrical imbalance caused by the injury, apply magnets around the head and neck.

72. **Headaches/migraines:** Place the negative north pole magnets on the areas of the head that hurt the most. You can also place them over the occipital and trapezoid area. The face mask helps relax facial muscles and it can clear nasal problems such as sinusitis or stress-related temporomandibular dysfunction (TMJ). The eye mask is also great for soothing frontal headaches and migraines because it blocks light from the eyes. Magnetic massages are excellent for helping the area relax and release toxins that tend to accumulate in face, neck and shoulder muscles.

73. **Hearing problems:** Depending on the cause, and as long as there's no infection present, I recommend applying the negative north pole to strengthen the eardrum. Apply it for thirty minutes, followed by a second thirty-minute session with the positive south pole. You can also use a wrap to secure a domino-shaped magnet in place.

74. **Heart disease/chest angina (angina pectoris):** Do not use this technique if you have a pacemaker. In cases of heart weakening, the heart muscles could weaken also, resulting in murmurs or reduced heart rate. In these cases, I recommend applying the positive south pole for ten minutes twice a day, preferably in the mornings and evenings, to improve the weakened heart valves. To treat chest angina and normalize cardiac irregularities like tachycardia, palpitations and arrhythmia, you can use a low power (400 to 700 gauss) negative north pole magnet, like a flex pad. I also suggest holding a cylinder magnet on the right hand. I recommend you wear a magnetic bracelet made with negative north pole polarity to control abnormal beatings of the heart and to soothe the right arm. Magnets can have positive effects on the circulatory function, as well as the dilation of blood vessels, providing tissues with better oxygenation and reducing the adhesiveness of blood and platelets. Magnetic therapy can also help undo other blockages in different parts of the body, such as arteries in the lower extremities, neck, and the blood vessels in

hands and arms. This therapy can prevent or improve cardiac conditions such as ischemic heart disease, angina pectoris and heart failure.

75. **Heel spurs:** I recommend the use of negative north pole magnetic insoles, meta-arch pads and magnetic ankle bracelets. I also suggest stretching the Achilles tendon and the other tendons that make up your foot.

76. **Hemorrhoids:** I suggest you place a negative north pole magnet, preferably strong like an N-1 or N-2 under you when you sit or lie down. It needs to be a strong magnet so that the therapeutic effect can reach the rectum, colon and abdomen.

77. **Herpes:** Viral infections such as this one can be a result of a weakened immune system. I suggest washing the affected area with water magnetized with the negative north pole for one hour twice a day. Drink water of the same polarity.

78. **Hiatal hernia:** The stress or stomach acidity you feel can start to travel upwards, mimicking a mini heart attack. To relief the pain and irritation this causes, place the negative north pole of a pillow or flexible magnetic support over the inferior part of the esophagus and over the upper part of your stomach while you're in a reclined position. If you have a pacemaker, do not use this technique if you have a pacemaker. I also recommend you drink water magnetized with the negative north pole.

79. **Hiccups:** To treat the sudden and repetitive contractions in the diaphragm I suggest you put a magnet over the stomach and then sleep over a magnetic pillow positioned around the T9 and T10 vertebrae.

80. **High cholesterol and triglycerides:** I recommend applying magnets to the entire body to promote integral blood circulation. Negative alkaline energy acts against fatty acids, neutralizing the negative or positive magnetic imbalance in the blood. Which is why it's beneficial to apply magnets during the day and at night. Making changes in your diet and drinking an abundant amount of polarized water is also encouraged.

81. **Hyperactivity:** Hyperactivity, attention deficit and other be-havioral problems in children may in part be related to nutri-tion (excess sugar), family situations, traumatic events, toxins in immunizations, the need for glasses, traumatic childbirth, among others. It's important that a chiropractic doctor evalu-ates them. The use of magnets has prove to be beneficial for children in any situation. I suggest you apply the negative north pole magnets to the child, they can lie on top of them or they can use a magnetic pillow. Positioning a negative north pole magnetic band over their forehead and temporal bones during the day and before going to sleep can help the child relax. In se-vere cases, this application is recommended three times a day for thirty to sixty minute sessions. The negative north pole has calming benefits that will help soothe the brain's nerve impulses and help oxygenate the blood.

82. **Hypertension:** For high blood pressure I suggest you use the negative north pole over the sternum and a positive south pole magnet on the upper part of the back, specifically around T2 and T3 for twenty to thirty minutes. I also recommend the daily use of a negative north pole magnetic neck band that can move to-wards the right side of the neck and a negative north pole mag-netic bracelet on the right wrist. You can compliment your ther-apy by sleeping on top of the magnets or a negative north pole magnetic pillow. Drinking water polarized with the negative north pole never hurts. Applying the negative north pole on the upper back area for twenty minutes can help reduce blood pres-sure. I also suggest you create a habit of measuring your blood pressure after each application to compare and evaluate results. You can use flexible magnets or shoulder pads with an additional negative north domino shaped magnet on the front side. Place the negative north pole N-1 or even N-2 on the back over the kidney area, alternating between right and left. You can also po-sition a magnetic back brace a little above the waist.

83. **Hyperthyroidism:** Use the negative north pole of the N-1 under your pillow, neckband or wear the negative north pole necklace.

I also recommend you drink water magnetized with the negative north pole. You can place the negative north pole in the palm of the left hand and under the right foot, while you place the positive south pole of the magnet in the palm of the right hand and under the left foot for ten minutes a day in the morning. This habit energizes the meridians.

84. **Hypoglycemia:** I suggest drinking polarized water daily and, once a week, drink water that's been polarized with the south positive pole. Wearing magnetic jewelry will soothe the symptoms associated with this condition.

85. **Hypotension:** To treat low blood pressure, I suggest a negative north pole magnetic neck band, turned to the left side of the neck, and a negative north pole magnetic bracelet on the left wrist. Use both daily. Sleep with a negative north pole magnet tucked under the pillow and drink water of the same polarity (alternating between two to three with glasses of water magnetized with the positive south pole during the week.) Monitor regularly your blood pressure levels. Adjust and take days off of magnetic therapy as you see necessary. Evaluate your situation and if you see it fit, restart therapy. To prevent vertigo associated with hypotension, I recommend holding a magnetic cylinder with your left hand. It's also important that you evaluate if this reaction can be related to any prescribed medication for hypertension or other chemical treatments. In these cases, magnetic therapy should include direct treatment of the adrenal and thyroid glands through ceramic magnets and the magnetic neck band.

86. **Hypothyroidism:** Before performing any type of magnetic therapy you should go through a blood analysis to evaluate your thyroid gland and determine the cause of the hypothyroidism. I recommend you stimulate your thyroid hormones. You can achieve this by applying a domino shaped magnet to the frontal part of your neck, just above the clavicle for thirty minutes, once or twice a day. Turn the domino magnet towards the positive south pole for twenty to thirty minutes and then go back to

the negative north pole for the same amount of time. Wear a magnetic necklace daily that is magnetized with both poles. Apply the negative north pole to the palm of the left hand and under the right foot, and the positive south pole of the magnet to the palm of the right hand and under the left foot for ten minutes a day in the morning. Drink water magnetized with the negative north pole and alternate poles using the magnetic pencil. If there's swelling, apply the negative north pole of the domino shaped magnet to the area for fifteen minutes on each side. Compliment that with a negative north pole magnetic necklace you wear daily. Avoid necklaces with both polarities made out of pearls or hematite until the swelling subsides. The effectiveness of this therapy depends on the intensity of the hypothyroidism.

87. **Impotence:** Apply a positive south pole magnet to the pubic region.

88. **Influenza:** Drink plenty of polarized water to hydrate and relief symptoms. Sleep with magnets to help ease body aches and restore your system.

89. **Insect bites:** Apply the negative north pole to the affected area for at least three hours to reduce pain and neutralize acidity. Wash the area with water magnetized with the negative north pole.

90. **Insomnia/sleep:** Magnetic therapy, both static and pulsed, has proven to have positive effects on circulating circadian rhythms and it also soothes the brain. Sleep patterns can be affected by the high frequency contamination of present electromagnetic fields from, like Wi-Fi. I recommend incorporating a north negative pole magnetic bracelet to your daily routine. I also suggest you apply a magnet of this same polarity to the space between your eyebrows for ten to twenty minutes. This consistent practice will stimulate the pineal gland, and promote relaxation. Placing a magnet on the bed but under your body will help reduce stress and muscle tensions, which will help you rest easier! The magnetic neckband is also very useful for improving sleep quality. Pulsating electromagnetic field therapy programs with specific low frequencies and reduced intensity, can soothe the nervous

system and promote rest. Delta frequencies set at 7 Hz are optional and can be customized according to your needs. Complement all this with herbal teas and homeopathic supplements. Chiropractic care and daily breathing exercises such as those employed in yoga, tai chi o Qi-gong can also contribute an improved quality of sleep. I suggest combining all these practices to obtain quicker results.

91. **Jet lag:** To reduce the symptoms take magnets with you on the plane, specially in the shape of magnetic jewelry or magnetic travel pillows. Drink polarized water and make use of your magnets as soon as you can after your travels.

92. **Joint implants:** Magnetic therapy, both static and pulsed, has been shown to have a positive impact on bone healing. It reduces inflammation and strengthens the bone around the damaged joints or implants. I suggest you consider this therapy even before going into surgery, because it might stimulate the bone and prepare it for the surgical procedure. Even cases with irreparable damages may see improvement thanks to the consistent use of magnetic knee braces and bands or N-1 ceramic magnets, 2" x 6" in preparation for surgery. This joint and body preparation process strengthens the area and reduces damage to the joint capsule. After surgery, continue your magnetic therapy regime. Use magnetic knee pads or N-1 negative north pole magnets to encourage recovery. I also recommend considering the use of magnets in cases of osteopenia before it develops into osteoporosis.

93. **Keloid (scar tissue):** Apply the negative north pole for thirty minutes, followed by the positive south pole for fifteen minutes.

94. **Knee pain:** I suggest you apply the negative north pole over the affected zone. Use magnetic knee pads or negative north pole magnets. You should be careful with your recovery process if it's a sport injury. You might feel better quicker, but that doesn't mean you've completed the healing process. You have to allow

the injury to heal completely before going back to your regular sports routine.

95. **Laryngitis:** I suggest you apply the negative north pole to the affected area, specially if it's infected. The magnetic neckband of the same polarity should be placed in the frontal part of the throat and it can be amplified with a doming shaped magnet. Practice this technique continuously to see better results. You can also gargle water magnetized with the negative north pole.

96. **Learning disabilities:** Apply a negative north pole magnet to the forehead and to the back of the head to promote relaxation, alertness and improved memory. I recommend using a magnetic pad and placing a negative north pole magnet under the pillow. You may also apply magnets to each temple for thirty to sixty minutes daily for three days, and then place it at the base of the skull. Keep the magnet in place as consistently as possible. You can also energize the meridians by placing the negative north pole magnet in the left palm and under the right foot, and the positive south pole magnet in the right palm and under the left foot for ten minutes each morning. Drink water magnetized with the negative north pole and follow the hyperactivity protocol in this guide.

97. **Liver disease:** This condition requires diagnosis and treatment by a specialist. You can compliment that treatment with magnetic therapy. You can also find more information about this condition in Sierra's and Davis letters. For liver-related problems, I suggest applying the negative north pole to the upper right side of the abdomen, under the rib cage, directly over the liver. I recommend you do it for thirty to forty five minutes three times a day. In more advanced cases, twice a day can work as well. Once you feel improvement, you can go down to thirty minutes in the morning and at night. Try to sleep with a magnetic cushion as much as you can, it's extremely beneficial. You can also sleep on top of the magnets.

98. **Lupus erythematosus:** Full body magnetic therapy using the negative north pole is recommended. Place N-1 or N-2 magnets

under the knees, on the back, and under your pillow at night. Hold the negative north pole in your left hand and place it under your right foot, while placing the positive south pole in your right hand and under your left foot for ten minutes daily to stimulate meridian points. Use PEMF therapy and drink water magnetized with the negative north pole. Refer also to the autoimmune disease section of this guide.

99. **Lyme disease:** Because of your condition, I initially suggest you visit a specialist. I recommend you go to the Fibromyalgia and autoimmune sickness sections, such as heart, kidneys, liver and arthritis. The combination of pulsating and static magnetic therapy will decrease inflammation, better your functions, relief your symptoms and promote healing within the body.

100. **Macular degeneration:** I suggest placing the negative north pole between the eyes for ten minutes for three times a day. Compliment this treatment by wearing the negative north pole magnetic eye mask at night or for short period of time during the day. I also recommend drinking water magnetized with the negative north pole.

101. **Magnetic deficiency syndrome:** The ideal treatment for this condition involves full-body exposure using a negative north pole magnetic bed. This promotes deep relaxation, reduces stress, enhances sleep quality, and helps the body restore its energetic balance. I also recommend treating the pineal gland regularly with a magnetic headband. Treat at least three hours a day.

102. **Multiple sclerosis:** Sleep over magnets or a negative north pole magnetic pillow. This will help you affront this condition. My suggestion is to hold a magnetic cylinder on your hand for fifteen minutes twice a day. I also recommend that you put a cylinder on the floor and, with bare feet, roll the cylinder back and forward. Make use of magnetic pillows, drink polarized water and apply magnets to the affected areas.

103. **Muscle spasms, muscle strains and sprains and joint pains:** Magnetic therapy significantly reduces muscular spasms.

Wearing a magnetic back brace, bands, flexible magnetic pads, or negative north pole magnets in specific areas will help with discomfort. Place a magnetic pad on the sacral area and sit or lie down. Magnetic application on the energetic meridians activates the flow of energy. For example, the bladder meridian, which crosses the sacrum, controls the energy flowing through the muscles of the back, including the shoulders. Increasing the flow of energy in the bladder area can relieve muscle problems and tensions that run down to the shoulders. For a torn muscle I suggest applying a negative north pole magnet, covering the area with a large magnetic pad or a magnetic strip. This will significantly relieve pain, reduce discomfort and reduce bruising around the tissue. I recommend placing magnets over the spasm as long as necessary. If you spend too much time sitting down at work, a magnetic cushion for your seat would be of great benefit, and if you need lumbar support you can try with a cushion contoured with magnets. You can use the magnets for several hours and then take a break, as you can wear the magnet all day and remove it at night or vice versa, as it's a common practice. You can have them on all the time and you can make exceptions when taking a shower. As soon as you're done, put them on again immediately. This rule also applies to joint pain. You can place a magnet over the desired joint for a period of time. By positioning the magnets on the corresponding acupuncture points you can also unlock a range of extra benefits. For leg cramps, I recommend you use negative north pole magnetic insoles and add calcium supplements to your diet. Wearing magnetic jewelry will also help you manage tension to prevent muscle spasms. You can also try applying the positive south pole to the area to relax the muscle contraction and then apply the negative north pole. Keep in mind that muscle strains or spasms are rarely the primary condition and are usually the result of an underlying pathology.

104. **Nausea:** Apply the negative north pole magnetic band over the upper abdomen, covering the stomach, liver, and gallbladder for thirty to sixty minutes or until relief is felt. You may also apply the magnet to the inside of your wrist, about two inches above

the crease at point PC-6 (pericardial meridian), or on the back of the neck. Drink water magnetized with the negative north pole.

105. **Nervousness:** Lie on a negative north pole magnetic pillow while holding a magnetic cylinder in your right hand. Use the magnetic headband or eye mask to help you relax. Stay in this position until you feel calm. Drink polarized water as part of your routine.

106. **Neuritis/Neuralgia:** Apply the negative north pole to the affected area to reduce pain and inflammation. Choose magnet size according to the location of the affected nerve. Lie on a negative north pole magnetic pillow or pad to relax the nervous system. To encourage nerve regeneration, place a negative north pole magnet two inches above the area and a positive south pole two inches below. This protocol may not show immediate results, but you will see benefits in the long run. If swelling occurs, remove the positive south pole and continue only with the negative north pole until symptoms improve. Use static magnets and PEMF therapy along the spine for systemic support. Drink plenty of magnetized water and take sublingual vitamin B-12.

107. **Obesity:** Use full-body magnets to stimulate blood flow. Begin by applying the positive south pole over the colon for ten minutes, three to four times a day, then immediately switch to the negative north pole for ten minutes or more. Then, immediately switch to the magnet's negative north pole on the colon for ten minutes or more. The entry of negative (alkaline) energy into the body helps dissolve fat deposits. Place negative magnets in belts over the abdominal fat. This area is associated with significant production of inflammatory molecules. Using magnets continuously during the day and night is beneficial because it reduces the inflammatory molecules circulating through the body, which affects the brain and the rest of the organism. This will help manage the lack of energy and motivation to engage in physical activity. In addition to magnetic therapy, I recommend the use of supports (wraps) and magnetic jewelry. It is essential to implement dietary

changes, adopt proper nutrition, modify behavior, increase physical activity, and drink magnetized water with the negative north pole, six to eight glasses of water a day. All of these steps combined over an extended period can contribute to treating obesity in a comprehensive way.

108. **Osteopenia/Osteoporosis:** Make sure your condition has been diagnosed by a specialist before you begin with this treatment. Both diseases involve decreased bone mineral density due to various causes. They may stem from the use of steroids, being bedridden, chemotherapy, celiac disease, autoimmune and inflammatory diseases, excessive consumption of cigarettes and alcohol, genetic factors, hyperthyroidism, diabetes, the use of antacids containing aluminum, among others. Apply magnets throughout the body and use a negative north pole magnetic pad on the shoulder, spine, or hips during daily activities. PEMF therapy is essential, and magnetic jewelry is also recommended. Drink six to eight glasses of water magnetized with the negative north pole daily.

109. **Pancreas:** Apply 4" x 6" N-2 magnets with the negative north pole over the epigastric region for thirty to sixty minutes twice a day. If insulin production is an issue, apply a positive south pole magnet for thirty minutes in the morning and at night.

110. **Parathyroid glands:** Research indicates that inflammation in the parathyroid glands and thyroids can be gradually stopped through exposure to biomagnetic energy (Davis, 1989). For the parathyroid glands, I recommend placing the negative north pole against the sides of the neck for fifteen minutes. If this discomfort isn't due to an infection, you can apply the positive south pole to the neck for fifteen minutes a day. This will control the amount of calcium in the blood. If the calcium isn't controlled, the negative north pole reduces and levels the calcium production within joints and fingers, decreasing the likelihood of developing arthritis.

111. **Parkinson's disease (PD):** I suggest you include chiropractic sessions to your routine to release the nervous system and stimulate constantly the cerebrospinal fluid. This illness affects the function of vital nerve cells and neurons in the brain, mainly in an area of the brain called substantia nigra. To treat this I recommend the use of static and pulsating magnetic therapy to the affected area. I suggest a high frequency full body pillow to stimulate the brain, nerves and abdomen. Also, placing negative north pole N-1 magnets under the pillow and feet will help promote good circulation. I recommend PEMF therapy for thirty minutes twice a day along with other treatments I've recommended in this section. It's important to highlight that static magnet and PEMF therapy has been a valuable contribution to the technology that treats Parkinson' disease, and it can help reduce and delay the progression of the disease.

112. **Pediatric diseases:** To treat chicken pox, mumps, measles and other similar childhood conditions you assist the child in using their magnets correctly. Instruct them to sleep on the magnets and polarize water for them to drink. As for infections, treatment is focused on the negative north pole. Magnets will help symptoms subside.

113. **Pleurisy and pneumonia:** I recommend applying magnetic therapy with negative north pole ceramic magnets directly over the area where you feel pain. Sleep on top of an N-1 or N-2 negative north pole magnet and drink plenty of polarized water.

114. **Post-Polio Syndrome:** Characterized by muscle pain and fatigue in individuals who had polio, this condition may improve with the application of negative north pole magnets directly to painful areas. Magnetic knee or ankle braces can help relieve discomfort. Sleep on an N-1 or N-2 magnet and drink polarized water regularly. In cases of muscle weakness without pain, multi-polar magnetic insoles may be beneficial.

115. **Prolapsed bladder or uterus:** Sit on a positive south pole magnetic cushion two or three times a day for thirty minutes. Magnetic back braces directed toward the lower abdomen can help

strengthen and support the bladder and uterine muscles when used with alternating polarities. This practice can help prevent relapses.

116. **Prostate:** For prostatitis or inflammation of the prostate, sit on a negative north pole N-2 ceramic magnet to relieve pain and reduce swelling. If no infection or inflammation is present, you can use the positive south pole for thirty minutes once or twice daily to promote prostatic fluid production. This can yield results within a few days. In cases of prostate cancer, only use the negative north pole, and sit on it for at least three to five hours daily. Drink six to eight glasses of water magnetized with the negative north pole.

117. **Raynauds disease:** I recommend placing the negative north pole on the wrists, the use of negative north pole magnetic insoles inside your shoes and drinking water magnetized with the negative north pole or both poles.

118. **Renal problems:** For pain, swelling, or pus in the back due to kidney issues, apply N-1 or N-2 ceramic magnets directly over the kidneys. Use the negative north pole for forty minutes to an hour, once or twice daily. With consistent use, this can help relieve symptoms over time and even improve the clarity of urine. The duration of treatment will vary depending on the case.

119. **Rheumatoid arthritis:** To address this chronic inflammatory condition, I suggest you place the negative north pole on the wrists and any other joint that is inflamed or in pain. Sleep with these supports on the affected areas or use a negative north pole magnetic pad. Use negative north pole magnetic insoles inside your shoes. It's also recommended that you drink water magnetized with the negative north pole and positive south pole. You can also refer to the Arthritis and Autoimmune Diseases sections of this book.

120. **Ringworm:** I suggest you position the negative north pole over the affected zone. You can also use small or flexible magnets. I also suggest you wash the zone with water magnetized with the

negative north pole and drink six to eight cups of water of the same polarity.

121. **Scar treatment:** Magnetic therapy can aid in scar healing. Place the negative north pole magnet over the affected area and drink and wash with water magnetized with the same polarity.

122. **Sciatica:** To treat this nerve pain that irradiates from the lower back area to the leg, I recommend placing a negative north pole magnet in each painful spot. I suggest the use of a magnetic insoles to attract the pain downwards, and the positive south pole on the soles can also be beneficial. Massage the buttock and calve with magnetic muscular simulators to release the sciatic nerve compression.

123. **Scleroderma:** For this complex disease which contains a significant autoimmune component I recommend the use of static and pulsating magnetic therapy to reduce inflammation, repair damaged tissue, halt disease progression and balance immune system functions. Treatment on the hands and feet is also beneficial.

124. **Scoliosis:** I suggest the use of magnets to help the muscles relax and contract, depending on the convex or concave side of the back curvature. The positive south pole is used to release tense muscles, while the negative north pole contracts muscles. I recommend a thirty minute daily treatment with two N-1 magnets, applying one pole at the time. The elastic band can be used to hold the magnets. I suggest you have a companion that can assist you with the placement of the magnets.

125. **Sexual impulse:** Dr. Sierra's investigations into magnetism demonstrated that sitting on a positive south pole increases sexual desire, while sitting on a negative north pole reduces it. Conduct your own investigation starting with twenty minute intervals. Use the N-1 with the correct polarity.

126. **Shingles:** I suggest applying ceramic magnets to the front and back of the body around nerve endings if the rash affects the chest area where the ribs are located. If the rash is on the face, I recommend placing ceramic magnets on the affected area for at

least three hours a day or as often as necessary to relieve symptoms. I recommend pressing gauze or cotton balls soaked in apple cider vinegar diluted with water magnetized with the negative north pole two to three times a day. I've seen the skin heal without scarring thanks to this treatment. Have your chiropractor give you an adjustment to reduce or alleviate the pain caused by intercostal neuritis. Supplement your treatment with sublingual vitamin B-12.

127. **Shoulder injury/rotator cuff syndrome:** Wear a shoulder brace magnetized with north negative pole energy or place the negative north pole directly over the area to relieve pain. The positive south pole can be used to stimulate circulation. Drink six to eight glasses of water magnetized with the negative north pole and complement the treatment with static and pulsating magnetic therapy.

128. **Shoulder tension:** Tension in the shoulders due to stress or posture can be addressed using a magnetic shoulder bib embedded with negative north pole magnets. This cushion wraps around the upper shoulders and provides localized relief. Wearing a magnetic bracelet daily helps keep pain under control. Add daily stretching and breathing exercises to further reduce tension.

129. **Sickle cell disease (SCD):** The objective here is to better oxygenation, decrease sedimentation of abnormal red blood cells, reduce the risk of infection, reduce any associated inflammation and assist the tissue through the recovery process through magnetic therapy. Because the entire vascular system is involved, I recommend PEMF therapy on the entire body. It's unwise to expect PEMF therapy to reverse sickle cell disease completely, but it has been found to be a useful treatment, especially when managing the associated pain.

130. **Sinus issues:** A magnetic face mask that covers the entire sinus area can offer great relief from sinus discomfort and pressure. Apply it as often as needed. For additional benefit, use a magnetic neckband and a facial magnetic massager.

131. **Skin:** For eczema, acne, and psoriasis, apply the negative north pole to the affected areas. You may use a thin cotton or linen cloth between the magnet and skin. Apply for thirty minutes once or twice a day. Magnetic therapy also benefits surrounding tissue.

132. **Sore throat, tonsillitis:** For throat pain and tonsillitis use Dr. Sierra's magnetic neckband. I recommend placing it with the negative north pole towards the throat, even in cases of infection. If one or both glands are throbbing from discomfort add the magnetic necklace and a domino shaped magnet and place both magnets over the gland that hurts. If you do not have an infection but you have a sore throat, I suggest applying the positive south pole of the domino shaped magnet for fifteen to twenty minutes. I also suggest you drink polarized water.

133. **Spinal cord injury:** This condition causes pain, affects the overall vitality of the tissues below the injury level and creates functional problems in organs because they're not receiving adequate nerve support in the spinal cord. This happens because when you sit for a long time the body exerts pressure on the organs. Not moving your body actively and experiencing many mood swings also adds to the problem. My experience with this condition comes from watching my dad, Dr. Sierra, treat a 30-year-old patient with a spinal cord injury. Dr. Sierra also advised her to put magnets on the back and cushion of her chair, along with her armrests and under her feet when receiving biomagnetic therapy, so she could receive magnetic therapy continuously. The patient didn't experience other complications from her condition and went on to live a full life. It's important that you have someone with you to assist you with the placement of the magnets if you're going to follow these recommendations.

134. **Sprain or strain:** Position the negative north pole directly on the affected area to treat the pain. You can move the magnet around the area, about two or three inches away to reduce pain and inflammation. Use the magnets continuously to see better results. You can find more information in the Bones and joints section of this guide.

135. **Surgery:** Before submitting yourself to surgery use magnets twenty four to forty eight hours before the procedure on the incision area. This can result in a more effective recovery period. The continued use of magnets over a wound after it's been sutured can accelerate the healing process. (Post-Surgery Recovery and Rehabilitation | www.neomedinstitute.com, n.d.).

136. **Swollen ankles:** Apply a negative north pole magnet to the kidney area to help stimulate urine production and reduce fluid retention. You can also use AccuPoint magnets directly on the swollen areas of the ankles to help decrease inflammation. Be sure to drink plenty of water magnetized with the negative north pole.

137. **Teeth and gums:** Exposing your teeth to a magnet for thirty minutes twice a day has proven to reduce, stop and even eliminate any pain that may be caused by nerves pressure, tissue inflammation, organ problems or fractures in the affected area of the body. It's been reported that for specific dental problems such as cavities, infected gums or roots, swelling, pus accumulations, soft gums and loose teeth, applying a magnet for thirty to forty minutes twice a day provides benefits. This can be achieved by using a wrap or a magnetic face mask. Pain usually subsides after three or four applications, swellings are reduced in two days and loose teeth can take several weeks to improve depending on the condition and cause. To relieve toothache, I recommend placing the negative north pole continuously on the affected area (cheek) and supplementing this treatment with gargling water magnetized with the negative north pole. It's important to keep in mind that the negative north pole may require greater depth for proper penetration if placed on ice.

138. **Tennis elbow (lateral epicondylitis):** For tennis elbow I recommend constantly using the magnetic band until the pain disappears. You can also prevent tennis elbow by using this same band, avoiding getting too close to the rib cage. It's very beneficial. Before and after playing tennis I recommend applying the

magnetic treatment to your elbow for thirty minutes daily for six weeks, followed by thirty minutes daily for four weeks.

139. **Tinnitus:** Apply the negative north pole of a domino-shaped magnet to the upper part of the affected ear. Sleep with an N-1 ceramic magnet under your pillow. This combination can help relieve symptoms. In more complex cases, consider evaluating other contributing factors, such as dental metal fillings. Drinking plenty of polarized water is also recommended.

140. **TMJ (temporomandibular joint):** For jaw pain commonly caused by teeth grinding, the discomfort typically occurs near the frontal earlobe, where the strongest muscle in the body is located. I recommend visiting a chiropractor for an adjustment and a gentle massage of the joint using the fingers or, ideally, a magnetic-tipped massager such as a negative north pole magnetic massager. You can also apply a small domino-shaped ceramic magnet with the negative north pole facing the skin for thirty minutes, three to four times a day, or until the pain subsides. You may hold the magnet in place or use 2,500-gauss magnetic dots for two to three hours twice daily. I also suggest using a magnetic neckband, as the jaw muscles extend into the neck area. The magnetic facial mask can help by covering most of the facial muscles. Consider massaging this joint preventively, especially after dental visits, as those appointments often cause significant emotional stress. Treating this joint gently and consistently helps prevent more serious complications.

141. **Tumors:** To help halt tumor growth or even dissolve them, apply negative north pole energy for thirty to forty minutes over the affected area twice a day. Results will vary depending on the type, size, and progression of the tumor. Benign tumors should also be treated directly with the negative north pole. Sleep over ceramic magnets of the same polarity and drink water magnetized with the negative north pole.

142. **Ulcer:** Use a domino-shaped magnet or a flexible magnetic strip with the negative north pole to relieve discomfort and support

tissue regeneration. Refer to the gastrointestinal disorders section for related guidance, such as swishing, gargling, and drinking water magnetized with the negative north pole. Always wash the affected area with water of the same polarity.

143. **Urinary problems, incontinence:** See the Bladder/Kidney section.

144. **Varicose veins/phlebitis:** Wear magnetic ankle braces or bands with the negative north pole. If swelling occurs near the knee, use a supportive knee brace that does not compress the area, as too much pressure can worsen swelling. Drink plenty of polarized water. You may also place 2,500-gauss magnetic points directly over the sore veins or capillaries until relief is achieved.

145. **Vertigo:** Magnetic application will depend on the root cause. If vertigo stems from the ear, place a negative north pole magnet over the affected ear, securing it with a headphone if needed, for about thirty minutes during the day. If vertigo is linked to digestive issues, place the magnet over the stomach area. Additionally, drink four ounces of water mixed with baking soda, stirred counterclockwise with a magnetic pencil to shift molecular polarity and improve absorption.

146. **Warts or skin lesions:** Apply a magnetic point directly over the wart or lesion and leave it overnight. Wash the area with water magnetized with the negative north pole and follow by drinking water of the same polarity.

147. **Whiplash:** In cases of cervical trauma, use the magnetic neck brace with the negative north pole placed at the base of the skull. Begin using it immediately and wear it throughout the day, even while sleeping if possible. Alternatively, use a negative north pole magnetic necklace daily. Seek chiropractic care promptly, and apply both ice and magnetic therapy. A cervical-contour magnetic pillow can help reverse damage caused by rapid neck motion. For older injuries, consistent use of the magnetic neck band and cervical pillow is highly recommended.

148. **Wrinkles:** Use magnets for whole-body strengthening, not just the face. Apply Sierra's magnetic eye shields or facial mask for thirty minutes morning and evening (and optionally midday). Rinse your face with north-polarized water and apply a lotion polarized with the north pole. Sleeping with a magnet can further support cellular rejuvenation and youthful vitality.

Glossary

1. **AlNiCo:** A high-energy alloy composed of aluminum, nickel, iron, cobalt, and copper. While AlNiCo magnets are not commonly used in magnetotherapy due to their higher cost compared to ceramic magnets, I recommend them for use as hand cylinders during both static and pulsed magnetic therapy sessions.

2. **Alternating current (AC):** An electric current that reverses direction at regular intervals. This is the standard current used in most household electrical wiring.

3. **Applied Kinesiology:** A diagnostic technique that assesses the strength of specific muscles under varying conditions to determine imbalances and guide treatment decisions. It is often referred to as AK or muscle testing.

4. **Biomagnetic Pair (BP):** A therapeutic method developed by Mexican scientist Dr. Isaac Goiz Durán more than twenty-seven years ago. This technique uses paired magnets of moderate intensity applied to specific points on the body to neutralize dysfunctional bioelectric charges and restore balance to the biomagnetic system. The magnets, usually domino-shaped, are color-coded: red for the positive south pole and black for the negative north pole. The positive south pole is applied only briefly. This method is popular in parts of South America, especially in low-resource settings, and is often used as an alternative to antibiotics. While Jarrot and I are certified in this technique (after two weeks and 100 hours of training), we do not practice it, but we value being informed about available modalities.

5. **Biomagnetism:** The applied science that examines the effects of magnetic energy on living organisms, including plants, animals, and humans.

6. **Bipolar magnet:** A magnet that presents both poles, the negative north and the positive south, applied simultaneously. Also referred to as alternating poles, this term describes a magnetic field pattern that alternates impulses from the north and south poles. This can be created using permanent magnets arranged in alternating polarity or through PEMF (pulsed electromagnetic fields) in an oscillating wave pattern.

7. **Chi:** The formless energy that animates life. Chi is the vital force behind both voluntary and involuntary movement, including the internal oscillations of the body's organs.

8. **Curie Point:** The temperature at which a ferromagnetic material becomes paramagnetic (775°C for iron). Most magnets will permanently lose their magnetism if heated beyond a certain threshold (approximately 350°C for ceramic magnets). For this reason, magnets should not be exposed to extreme heat, such as being left in a hot car or under direct sun.

9. **Diamagnetism:** A property of materials in which the induced magnetic field opposes the applied magnetic field. All substances exhibit some degree of diamagnetism, which causes a weak repulsion from magnets.

10. **Direct current (DC):** An electric current that flows in a single, constant direction, such as that produced by batteries.

11. **Electromagnet:** A device made up of coils of wire wrapped around a core of soft or wrought iron. When electric current flows through the coils, a magnetic field is produced.

12. **Electromagnetic induction:** The generation of an electric current in a conductor resulting from a change in magnetic flux through the circuit.

13. **Electromagnetic radiation:** Emission generated by an electromagnetic field (EMF), which can affect the behavior of

nearby charged particles. Man-made EMFs, such as those from televisions, computers, and household appliances, can negatively impact human health. These fields are also called electromagnetic smog. It's important to distinguish passive and pulsed magnetic fields used in therapy from these artificial EMFs. Pulsed magnetic field therapy equipment transforms alternating current (AC) into direct current (DC), emitting controlled pulses at therapeutic frequencies. Battery-powered PEMF devices also operate using DC to produce these beneficial frequencies.

14. **Electromagnetism:** A branch of physics that studies the interactions between electric currents and magnetic fields. Electromagnetism is one of the fundamental forces of nature. It was first discovered by physicist Hans Christian Ørsted and further developed by scientists Michael Faraday and James Clerk Maxwell.

15. **Ferrimagnetism:** A form of magnetism found in ferrites: materials known for their high resistance and useful properties. Ferrites are commonly used in the cores of high-frequency transformers and in electronic components, including memory units in computers.

16. **Ferrite ceramic magnets:** A synthetic ceramic material composed of iron oxide combined with one or more metallic elements, such as strontium or barium ferrite. These magnets are ferrimagnetic, meaning they are attracted to magnetic fields and can become permanently magnetized. Though not as strong as neodymium magnets, ferrite magnets are highly durable, cost-effective, and ideal for therapeutic use. Thanks to the work of Davis & Sierra, these magnets are manufactured with a grade 8 rating and a gauss strength of 3,850 (with 1,300 gauss on the surface). They are specifically made with opposite poles (negative north pole on one side and a positive south pole on the other) to support healing. However, they are fragile and must be handled with care. If not dropped or mishandled, they can

be an important investment, retaining their strength for over sixty years.

17. **Ferromagnetic materials:** Substances that can be easily magnetized when placed within a magnetic field. Examples include iron, cobalt, and nickel.

18. **Ferromagnetism:** A property of certain materials, such as iron, nickel, and cobalt, that exhibit very high magnetic permeability and can retain magnetization even after the external magnetic field is removed.

19. **Flexible high intensity magnet:** A material made by combining dry ferrite powder with a rubber polymer resin, which can be magnetized. It is typically available in tape form with widths of one to three inches and thicknesses of 1/8 or 1/4 inch. The magnetic field has a negative north pole on one side and a positive south pole on the other. These magnets are the foundation of Dr. Sierra's well-known magnetic "magic bands."

20. **Galvanometer:** An instrument used to detect and measure low-intensity electric currents.

21. **Gamma:** A unit of measurement equal to one hundred-thousandth of a gauss. These waves are measured in cycles per second, which we describe as Hertz (Hz). This term is commonly used in geophysics to refer to variations in the Earth's magnetic field. Gamma values are used in geophysics to measure variations in the Earth's magnetic field. For example, magnetic storms may register at 40 to 50 gammas. The human heart produces a magnetic field of less than one gamma, muscles produce about one-tenth of a gamma, and brain neurons generate approximately one-hundredth of a gamma. The fastest brain waves are known as gamma waves.

22. **Gauss:** A unit of magnetic flux density or magnetic induction intensity, commonly used to describe magnetic force. Gauss is used to classify the strength of a magnet. One gauss is equal to 10^{-4} Tesla (T) in the International System of Units. The Earth's magnetic field measures approximately half a gauss. The unit

is named after 19th-century German scientist and mathematician Carl Friedrich Gauss.

23. **Induction lines:** Visual representations of the flow and motion of magnetic energy around a magnet, used to illustrate the direction and behavior of a magnetic field.

24. **Magnetic energy:** The energy stored within a magnetic field.

25. **Magnetic field deficiency syndrome:** A condition characterized by symptoms that arise from insufficient magnetic exposure in the human body. It is believed to result from the weakening of Earth's magnetic field and prolonged exposure to artificial electromagnetic environments.

26. **Magnetic field:** The area surrounding a magnet where its influence can be felt. This force field is generated by the motion of electric charges. The strength of a magnetic field is measured in Gauss (G) or Tesla (T).

27. **Magnetic force:** The attractive or repulsive force exerted by a magnet on other magnetic materials or moving charged particles. This is the force you feel when two magnets either pull together or push apart. Magnetic force is measured in gauss.

28. **Magnetic pole:** The point on Earth where magnetic meridians converge. There are two: the magnetic north and the magnetic south poles.

29. **Magnetic poles of a magnet:** All magnets have a negative north pole and a positive south pole. If you don't have a magnetometer, you can identify the poles manually: suspend a bar magnet or cylindrical magnet from its center using a string or wire, ensuring it swings freely away from other metallic objects. It will eventually align with Earth's magnetic field. Use a compass to determine which end points north. This end is the magnet's positive south pole, as opposite poles attract. Mark the identified side (usually red for south), and label the other accordingly. Remember, like poles repel and opposite poles attract.

30. **Magnetism:** A branch of physics that studies the properties and behaviors of magnets, whether natural or artificial, and the phenomena associated with them. Magnetism is commonly understood as an invisible physical force that acts on matter.

31. **Magnetite:** A naturally occurring magnetic mineral composed of iron oxide (Fe_3O_4), also classified as a ferromagnetic black spinel. It is sometimes called the magnetic stone. Legend has it that Queen Cleopatra wore a magnetite stone on her forehead, believing it would preserve her youth and beauty.

32. **Magnetization:** The process by which a material that previously exhibited no magnetic properties becomes magnetized through exposure to a magnetic field.

33. **Magnetometer:** An instrument used to measure and study variations in the Earth's magnetic energy. More broadly, the term refers to any device that measures the intensity of a magnetic field. Carl Friedrich Gauss significantly contributed to the development of the magnetometer in 1831. Magnetic field strength measured by this device is often expressed in Tesla units.

34. **Mesmerism:** An 18th-century theory proposing that all living beings are influenced by a "magnetic fluid" that can be redirected or concentrated through physical manipulation or passes. This concept was introduced by Franz Anton Mesmer.

35. **Modality:** A method or technique used in therapy or treatment.

36. **Negative north pole:** Also known as bionorth, this negative polarity is considered the "healing" side of a magnet. It is cooling, calming, and sedative; it reduces inflammation, slows down abnormal growth, detoxifies, and supports elimination. In Traditional Chinese Medicine (TCM), it corresponds to Yin, or negative polarity. It is commonly identified with white, blue, or green colors for therapeutic use.

37. **Neodymium magnets:** The most powerful type of permanent magnet, made from a combination of iron alloy, boron,

and the rare earth element neodymium. First produced in 1983, they are commonly referred to as neomagnets. These are often embedded in stainless steel or titanium magnetic jewelry and sometimes coated with resin for durability. They are also found in therapeutic body wraps. Always ensure that the negative north pole faces the skin.

38. **Oersted:** A unit of magnetic force used to measure the magnetizing strength applied to a material placed inside a current-carrying coil. It is symbolized by the letters Oe or B and named after scientist Hans Christian Ørsted.

39. **Paramagnetism:** A material property whereby a substance becomes magnetized in the same direction as an applied magnetic field, though with significantly less intensity than ferromagnetic materials.

40. **Permanent magnet:** A magnet that retains its magnetism without requiring a continuous electric current. This occurs because some of the electrons within the iron atoms remain aligned in their spin direction. Common materials used to create permanent magnets include iron oxide, samarium, cobalt, and neodymium.

41. **Polarity:** The characteristic of having two opposing poles (positive [south] and negative [north]) in a magnetic or electrical system.

42. **Polarized water:** Water that has been exposed to either the negative north pole or the positive south pole of a magnet. Water polarized with the negative north pole is suitable for human consumption, while water exposed to the positive south pole can be used for plants or other non-ingestible uses.

43. **Polarized:** Having both poles; synonymous with magnetized.

44. **Pole:** Each end of a magnet or an electric circuit.

45. **Positive south pole:** Also known as biosouth, this positive polarity stimulates warmth and activity. It promotes growth, builds up tissue, tones, strengthens, and supports accumulation.

In Traditional Chinese Medicine (TCM), it corresponds to Yang, or positive polarity. It is commonly marked with red for therapeutic identification.

46. **Solenoid:** A coil of conductive wire through which an electric current is passed, generating a magnetic field inside the coil. The magnetic field disappears when the current stops.

47. **Spins:** A concept from quantum mechanics that refers to the angular momentum of individual subatomic particles.

48. **Static magnetic therapy:** The application of unmoving (static) magnets to the body for health benefits. When used for therapeutic purposes, these are referred to as therapy magnets or biomagnets.

49. **Static magnets:** Stationary magnets that emit a direct current (DC) static magnetic field. These magnets provide several health benefits and are used to counteract the negative effects of electromagnetic pollution and to compensate for the reduction of Earth's magnetic field in the body.

50. **Tesla:** Tesla (T) is a measurement unit that describes magnetic flux density or magnetic force. The unit was named in 1960 after scientist and inventor Nikola Tesla. One Tesla is equivalent to 10,000 gauss.

51. **The figure 8:** A geometric illustration of energy movement that shows the complete separation of opposing charges or potentials at the ends of a magnetic bar or cylinder. At the center of the figure-eight lies a neutral zone known as Bloch's Wall, where opposing energies cancel each other out and electrons spin in opposite directions along the boundary.

References

Alberts B, Johnson A, Lewis J, et al. Molecular Biology of the Cell. 4th edition. New York: Garland Science; 2002. The Chemical Components of a Cell.
https://www.ncbi.nlm.nih.gov/books/NBK26883/

Becker, R. O., & Marino, A. A. (1982). Electromagnetism and life. Suny Press.

Casale, R., Alaa, L., Mallick, M., & Ring, H. (2009). Phantom limb related phenomena and their rehabilitation after lower limb amputation. European journal of physical and rehabilitation medicine, 45(4), 559–566.

CH, B. (1962). The direct current control system. A link between environment and organism. NY State J Med, 62, 1169-1176.

Charles F. Haanel (2017). The New Master Key System, p.320, Simon and Schuster

Cook, E.S., Smith, S.M.J. (1964). Increase of Trypsin Activity. In: Barnothy, M.F. (eds) Biological Effects of Magnetic Fields. Springer, Boston, MA.
https://doi.org/10.1007/978-1-4757-0214-9_23

Davis, A. R. (1989). The anatomy of biomagnetism.

NCI Dictionaries. (n.d.). National Cancer Institute.
https://www.cancer.gov/publications/dictionaries/cancer-terms/def/homeostasis

Electromagnetic fields and cancer. (2022, May 30). National Cancer Institute.
https://www.cancer.gov/about-cancer/causes-prevention/risk/radiation/electromagnetic-fields-fact-sheet#top

Faraday, Michael;Royal Society (Great Britain). (n.d.). On the magnetization of light and the illumination of magnetic lines. https://library.si.edu/digital-library/book/onmagnetizationo01-fara

Goodwin, T. J. (2006, January 1). An Optimization of Pulsed Electro-Magnetic Fields study. NASA Technical Reports Server (NTRS). https://ntrs.nasa.gov/citations/20070004785

July 1820: Oersted and electromagnetism. (n.d.). https://www.aps.org/publications/apsnews/200807/physicshistory.cfm

Matan. (2023, August 2). How does Faraday's Law work? Electricity - Magnetism. https://www.electricity-magnetism.org/how-does-faradays-law-work/

Montero Vega, V., Montero Campello, M., Sierra Figueredo, P., Sierra Figueredo, S., & Frómeta Jiménez de Castro, E. (2014). Mortalidad por infarto agudo de miocardio y su relación con las tormentas solares y geomagnéticas en la provincia Guantánamo. *Revista Cubana de Cardiología y Cirugía Cardiovascular, 20*(2), 78-83. https://revcardiologia.sld.cu/index.php/revcardiologia/article/view/516/586

Nakagawa, K. (1976). Magnetic Field Deficiency Syndrome and Magnetic Treatment. Japan Medical Journal, 2745. http://ddata.over-blog.com/xxxyyy/2/91/31/81/Champ-magnetique/761204-Mag.Field-Deficiency-Syndr.-Mag.Treatment.pdf

Pasek, J., Pasek, T., Sieroń A., et al. (2012). Magnetotherapy in the treatment of pain after limb amputation – Case report. BÓL, 13(1), 43.

Pirahanchi, Y., Jessu, R., & Aeddula, N. R. (2023, March 13). Physiology, Sodium potassium pump. StatPearls - NCBI Bookshelf. https://www.ncbi.nlm.nih.gov/books/NBK537088/

Power in a Magnet Part 1. Aug 2017. (n.d.). Health Magnetic Store & More | San Juan, Puerto Rico. https://www.energiamagnetica.com/videos/power-in-a-magnet?

srsltid=AfmBOopAj9v_uyvnrUlUe3e7ym-DZ7_muxb2_wb3L-NAK0aL6FumjJTR8

Schumann, W. O. (1952). Über die strahlungslosen Eigen-schwingungen einer leitenden Kugel, die von einer Luftschicht und einer Ionosphärenhülle umgeben ist. Zeitschrift für Natur-forschung A. 7 (2): 149–154. doi:10.1515/zna-1952-0202

Sisken, B., & Walker, J. (1995). Therapeutic aspects of electromag-netic fields for Soft-Tissue healing. https://www.semanticscholar.org/paper/Therapeutic-Aspects-of-Electromagnetic-Fields-for-Sisken-Walker/9a0b5a4c22f2902f414c7742e5fb3cf35527d64f

Skjærvø, G. R., Fossøy, F., & Røskaft, E. (2015). Solar activity at birth predicted infant survival and women's fertility in historical Norway. Proceedings of the Royal Society B: Biological Sciences, 282(1801), 20142032. https://doi.org/10.1098/rspb.2014.2032

Sotzny, F., Blanco, J., Capelli, E., Castro-Marrero, J., Steiner, S., Murovska, M., Scheibenbogen, C., & European Network on ME/CFS (EUROMENE) (2018). Myalgic Encephalomyelitis/Chronic Fatigue Syndrome - Evidence for an autoimmune dis-ease. Autoimmunity reviews, 17(6), 601–609. https://doi.org/10.1016/j.autrev.2018.01.009

The Editors of Encyclopaedia Britannica. (2024, February 13). Newton's law of gravitation | Definition, Formula, & Facts. Ency-clopedia Britannica. https://www.britannica.com/science/Newtons-law-of-gravita-tion

The Magnetic Blueprint of Life by Davis, Albert Roy. (n.d.). https://www.amazon.ca/Magnetic-Blueprint-Life-Albert-Davis/dp/0911311157

The Nobel Peace Prize 1962. (n.d.). NobelPrize.org. https://www.nobelprize.org/prizes/peace/1962/pauling/other-prize/

The Nobel Prize in Physics 1913. (n.d.). NobelPrize.org. https://www.nobelprize.org/prizes/physics/1913/onnes/facts/

The Nobel Prize in Physiology or Medicine 1931. (n.d.). Nobel-Prize.org. https://www.nobelprize.org/prizes/medicine/1931/warburg/biographical/

Universidad Finis Terrae. (n.d.). Química: Enlaces químicos. https://uft.cl/images/futuros_alumnos/profesores_orientadores/material-pedagogico/Guia_3_Enlaces_quimicos.pdf

Dr. Sierra's personal inspiration list

This list includes books and websites that were relevant to the author throughout the development of this book's contents, but are not explicitly mentioned in the text.

Beasley, V. R. (1979). *Your electro-vibratory body: A Study of the Life Force as Electro-vibratory Phenomena.* Dr Hills Technologies.

Becker, R. O. (1990). *Cross currents: The Promise of Electromedicine, the Perils of Electropollution.* Tarcher.

Becker, R., & Selden, G. (1998). *The body electric: Electromagnetism And The Foundation Of Life.* Harper Collins.

Dispenza, J. (2015). *You are the placebo: Making Your Mind Matter.* Hay House, Inc.

Dispenza, J. (2017). *Becoming supernatural: How Common People are Doing the Uncommon.* Hay House, Inc.

Francis, E. A. (2017). *The body heals itself: How Deeper Awareness of Your Muscles and Their Emotional Connection Can Help You Heal.* Llewellyn Worldwide.

Hay, L. (1995). *You can heal your life.* Hay House, Inc.

Jarrot Sierra, J. R. (2019). *Enfócate y cambia tu salud.*

Learn Qi Gong | Chi Gong | Holden QiGong. (2023, January 30). Holden QiGong. https://www.holdenqigong.com/

Lipton, B. H. (2015). *The biology of belief: Unleashing the Power of Consciousness, Matter & Miracles.*

Meyers, B. A. (2013). *PEMF - the fifth element of health: Learn Why Pulsed Electromagnetic Field (PEMF) Therapy Supercharges Your Health Like Nothing Else!* BalboaPress.

O'Bryan, T. (2016). *The autoimmune fix: How to Stop the Hidden Autoimmune Damage That Keeps You Sick, Fat, and Tired Before It Turns Into Disease.* Rodale Books.

O'Bryan, T. (2018). *You can fix your brain: Just 1 Hour a Week to the Best Memory, Productivity, and Sleep You've Ever Had.* Rodale Books.

Pawluk, W. (2021). *Supercharge Your Health with PEMF Therapy: How Pulsed Electromagnetic Field (PEMF) Therapy Can Jumpstart Your Health, Banish Pain, Improve Sleep, and Help Prevent and Relieve Over 80 Common Health Conditions.*

Sierra, I. (1970). *Power In A Magnet*

Sierra & Jarrot Quiropractica y Biomagnetismo. (n.d.). YouTube. https://www.youtube.com/@DrJorgeJarrot

Tolle, E. (2010). *The power of now: A Guide to Spiritual Enlightenment.* New World Library.

Villoldo, A. (2019). *Grow a new body: How Spirit and Power Plant Nutrients Can Transform Your Health.* Hay House, Inc.

Villoldo, A., & Villoldo, P. D. A. (2010). The four insights: Wisdom, Power, and Grace of the Earthkeepers. ReadHowYouWant.com.

About the Author

Dr. Irma I. Sierra, B.S, D.C., F.I.C.P.A.

Dr. Irma Sierra was born in San Juan, Puerto Rico, the daughter of Dr. Ralph U. Sierra and Irma Rivera Santiago. Her father, the first chiropractor in Puerto Rico, was instrumental in creating the law and the Board of Examiners that legalized the practice of chiropractic care on the island in 1952. He was also a renowned scientist and a pioneer in the use of biomagnetism in Puerto Rico.

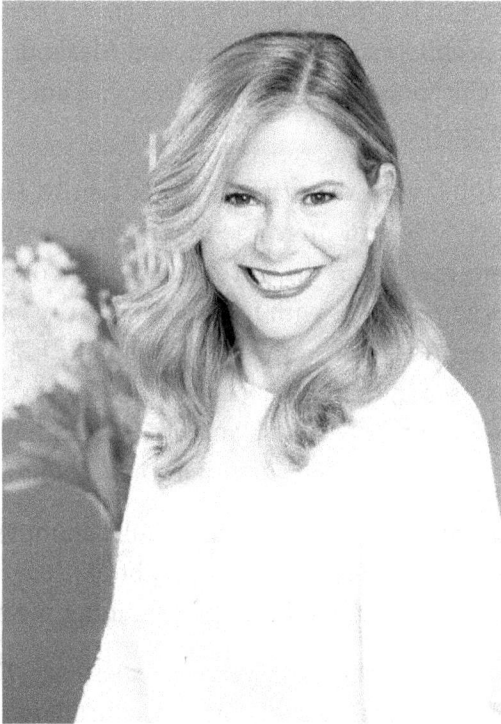

Growing up surrounded by science and discovery, Dr. Sierra worked alongside her father at his clinic, assisted in his laboratory, and accompanied him to local and international conferences. Chiropractic care and magnetic therapy have been part of her life from an early age, and she could not imagine a path that did not involve serving humanity through healing.

She earned her Doctor of Chiropractic degree from New York Chiropractic College in 1984. That same year, she became the first Puerto Rican woman to practice chiropractic care in Puerto Rico. Dr. Sierra also broke new ground as the first female president of both the *Junta Examinadora de Quiroprácticos de Puerto Rico* (Puerto Rico Board of Chiropractic Examiners) and the *Asociación de Quiroprácticos de Puerto Rico* (Puerto Rico Chiropractic Association), as well as the first female delegate to the *American Chiropractic Association* and the *Federation of Chiropractic Licensing Boards*. She is licensed to practice in New York and Florida.

In 1985, she founded *Clínica Quiropráctica Dra. Sierra* in San Juan. Ten years later, her husband, Dr. Jorge C. Jarrot, joined the clinic, and they renamed it *Clínica Quiropráctica Jarrot Sierra* with the hope that their three children, Jorge, Adrián, and Alexandra, would one day continue the chiropractic legacy. That dream became reality, as all three are now chiropractors.

In 2004, with the support of her family, Dr. Sierra founded *Health Magnetic Store & More*, the first magnetic product store in Puerto Rico. Concerned about the increasing number of poorly manufactured products and magnets with mislabeled polarity and strength on the market, she decided to offer the public the same high-quality magnetic products used in their clinical practice. Today, the store receives orders from around the world, and Dr. Sierra frequently exhibits her products at local and international conventions.

Committed to educating the public about the healing properties of magnets, she published her first book, *Power in a Magnet*, in 2007. It was later translated into Spanish under the title *El Poder del Imán*.

With over twenty-five years of experience, Dr. Sierra has not fully retired. She continues to work as a consultant at *Jarrot Sierra Chiropractic Clinic* and remains active in research and development for *Health Magnetic Store & More*. She also launched *Dr. Sierra's Naturals*, a line of more than thirty non-GMO supplements, free of gluten, corn, wheat, yeast, sugar, milk, eggs, starch, preservatives, and artificial colors. Additionally, she founded *Dr. Sierra Magnets*, a line of federally and state-registered magnetic products specifically designed for therapeutic use.

Throughout her career, Dr. Sierra has participated extensively in radio, television, and print media. She has conducted numerous lectures both locally and internationally on chiropractic care and biomagnetism. Currently, she co-hosts the educational television program *Tu Salud* alongside her husband and daughter, previously known as *Salud en Familia*. She also offers regular health and wellness lectures at her clinic, focusing on chiropractic care, nutrition, biomagnetism, and the benefits of natural healing practices.

Career Highlights:

1. 1984: Earned Doctor of Chiropractic degree

2. 1995: Obtained Pediatric Chiropractic Fellowship (F.I.C.P.A.)

3. 1998–2000: President of the *Asociación de Quiroprácticos de Puerto Rico*

4. 2002–2005: Member of the *Junta Examinadora de Quiroprácticos de Puerto Rico*

5. 2003–2007: Delegate of the *American Chiropractic Association* representing Puerto Rican chiropractors in Washington, D.C.

6. 2005–2009: President of the *Junta Examinadora de Quiroprácticos de Puerto Rico*

www.ingramcontent.com/pod-product-compliance
Lightning Source LLC
Chambersburg PA
CBHW070342270326
41926CB00017B/3943